Multiculturalism and the Therapeutic Process

Multiculturalism and the Therapeutic Process

JUDITH MISHNE

THE GUILFORD PRESS
New York   London

© 2002 The Guilford Press
A Division of Guilford Publications, Inc.
72 Spring Street, New York, NY 10012
www.guilford.com

Printed in the United States of America

Library of Congress Cataloging-in-Publication Data
available from the Publisher.

ISBN 1-57230-775-7

In memory of my father, Dr. Moses I. Marks, and in honor of my mother, Lillian K. Marks, who were my first role models and teachers about diversity. As clearly as if it were yesterday, I remember their acts of empathy, celebration, and joyful, loyal responsiveness to their multicultural circle of friends and colleagues. I consider myself fortunate to have grown up in a household enriched by my parents' lifelong cross-racial and cross-cultural friendships.

People talk to you a great deal about your education, but some good, sacred memory, preserved from childhood, is perhaps the best education.
—FYODOR DOSTOYEVSKY, "Epilogue,"
The Brothers Karamazov

About the Author

Judith Mishne, DSW, is a Full Professor at the Shirley M. Ehrenkranz School of Social Work, New York University, where she has been since 1979. She has published numerous texts, most recently, *The Evolution and Application of Clinical Theory: Perspectives from Four Psychologies* (1993, Free Press) and *The Learning Curve: Evaluating Children's Academic and Social Competence* (1996, Jason Aronson). She has edited three texts, is working on a fourth with colleagues, and has published numerous articles in various publications, in addition to over 100 professional presentations at conferences.

Dr. Mishne serves as consulting editor on the *Journal of Analytic Social Work* and the *Child and Adolescent Social Work Journal*. She has been a Visiting Scholar at the Bar Ilan University School of Social Work and at the University of Haifa School of Social Work, both in Israel. She also maintains a private practice.

Preface

We all have multiple cultural identities. As individuals, we live in a context of family, group, and community; in fact, we may have affiliations or memberships in a number of groups and communities related to our work, education, economics, special interests, and friendship circles. Each of us has varying levels of consciousness of our cultural identities, ranging from naiveté or lack of understanding to a sophisticated, multiperspective integration. Multicultural issues include language, gender, ethnicity/race, religion/spirituality, sexual orientation, age, physical issues, trauma, and socioeconomic realities. These variables commonly have a profound impact on a treatment relationship. This text aims to heighten clinicians' multicultural awareness and enhance their skills in working with a culturally diverse patient population. This will include ethnic sharing, valuing diversity, and making multiculturalism personal. The inner monologue of the clinician is also presented, since it reflects inferences, feelings, questions, and reservations, as well as countertransference responses, which often include cultural countertransference.

Lum (2000) notes that multicultural education has moved from exposure to ethnocultural intricacies, to goals of fairness, tolerance, prejudice reduction, and "support for the actualization of basic human rights. It includes professional training programs on stereotype and prejudice in one's own life, race relations and diversity workshops and culturally competent supervision" (p. 4). In keeping with these educational goals are principles of culturally competent practice with individuals, families, and groups that address all areas of diversity. Rounds, Weil, and Bishop (1994) offer four such principles, which are clearly demonstrated in the present text. Rounds and colleagues emphasize (1) acknowledgment and valuation of diversity, in terms of understanding how race, culture, and ethnicity contribute to the uniqueness of each individual, family, and community, as well as how diversity exists within each ethnic, cultural, and racial group; (2) a clinician's cultural self-assessment in regard to his or her own culture, and its impact on personal and professional beliefs and behaviors; (3) the acquisition of cultural awareness of each client's background; and (4) the adaptation of skills to the needs and styles of each client's culture.

This book aims to provide a clear and comprehensive presentation of the fundamentals of cross-cultural psychotherapy (i.e., psychotherapy in which the members of the therapeutic dyad are of different races and/or cultures). "Although it is critical for therapists to have a basic understanding of the culture-specific life values of different groups, there is the ever-present danger of over-generalizing and stereotyping" (Sue & Sue, 1990, p. 72). Concurring with this caution, I offer no generalizations in this book about clinical work with clients of color, and/or work with this or that specific ethnic, racial, or immigrant group. Instead, my approach is to discuss the treatment process and treatment relationship in the context of cross-cultural psychotherapy, and to use case material to illustrate different portions of the treatment process, as well as the various sorts of treatment issues and relationships that can and do occur.

I have chosen case material that represents a cross-section of highly intelligent and psychologically minded clients of various ages and various racial minority and immigrant groups, to challenge a dangerous bias within the mental health professions—namely, that people from such minority groups lack the capacity for self-reflection and are unable to explore the meaning of their experiences (Olarte & Lenz, 1984; Perez Foster, 1993). Because the treatment process with the selected clients reflects their capacities for insight and introspection, I have drawn on the psychoanalytic literature to demonstrate its usefulness. In fact, I consider a psychoanalytic perspective essential in clinical work with these clients.

The theoretical perspective includes changing models of psychoanalysis for the accommodation of diversity. Although references to and usages of drive theory and ego psychology are appropriate (especially in the discussions of assessment), self psychology, with its emphasis on empathy, and a relational model (i.e., object relations), which takes "account of the interaction of the intrapsychic organizations of each of the participants in an interaction, as well as the events taking place in the interpersonal field" (Altman, 1996, p. 198), are emphasized. Altman (1996) advocates the utility of a two-person (client and clinician) and/or three-person (client, clinician, and agency) clinical psychoanalytic model for taking account of race, class, and the impact of public culture. This widened lens prevents the clinician from relying only on superficial reflections of deeper unconscious conflict. Likewise, intersubjectivity theory examines the intersubjective field constituted by the reciprocal interplay between the two or more subjective worlds of client and clinician. This theory is viewed as a major advance in cross-cultural psychotherapy, and is presented in this text as another model for practice.

In addition to the conventional examination of transference and countertransference, culturally competent psychotherapy requires that clinicians "examine in an ongoing way, the following questions which relate to countertransference. Who am I? Who do others (particularly the client and family) think I am? What are my attitudes and beliefs—particularly about the client's racial ethnicity? The clinician should assess his or her own degree of biculturality" (Manoleas, 1996, p. 25). The foci described above are offered to assist clinicians in how they listen and finally hear what patients struggle to share. Ideally, the demonstrated communication process will enable clinicians in cross-cultural practice to engage an increasingly diverse client population with ease, understanding, and empathic, appropriate attention to cultural realities that are too often either ignored or viewed as marginal to psychodynamic theory and practice.

Moreover, Falicov (1998) emphasizes that a clinician should recognize and respect both the differences *and* the similarities in color, class, ethnicity, and/or gender between the clinician and the client. Such a perspective is mistakenly ignored by those practitioners who solely focus on issues of race, ethnicity, culture, and socioeconomic milieu that *differ* from their own. This results in emotionally charged biases about clinicians' own ethnic identities, and about those of their ethnic or racial "stranger" clients.

In this text, I offer self-disclosure about the reactions, actions, and feelings that my own cross-cultural work has aroused in me, in order to inform the reader about some of the hidden or forbidden agendas that commonly occur in the transferential–countertransferential exchange in a cross-cultural dyad. This inner monologue of inferences, feelings, questions, and reservations, I believe, reflects my own efforts to deal with the issues of cultural transference and countertransference in the ways described above. I concur with Perez Foster (1998b) that the "more disparate the cultural worlds of the therapeutic dyad, the more that the therapeutic enterprise needs to be taken as a joint quest for understanding and meaning, with the therapist needing to be particularly cautious about exercising his or her culturally circumscribed view of human behavior" (p. 168).

At the conclusion of this book, therefore, I hope that the reader will be able to see and feel the impact of culture and ethnicity on the treatment process and in the patient's life, and therefore on the evolution of the patient's cultural identity, which is integral to the formation of a cohesive self. As noted above, self psychology and intersubjectivity theory, with their emphasis on responsiveness, form the basis of the practice model presented. They have been selected because of their unique contributions to techniques of treatment: They facilitate rapport and strengthen patients' beliefs that they and their subjective worlds (indeed, their world views) can be understood by another. The resulting practice model facilitates bringing issues of culture, race, ethnicity, and class into the therapy room in a way that enhances the therapeutic relationship and thereby helps the clinician to avoid typical errors (such as ignoring a cultural focus, exhibiting culture- and/or color-blindness, or regarding race and ethnicity as only tangential to therapy). The emphasis on differences between therapists and their clients offers a more complete appreciation of a myriad of other crucial variables in the lives of clients (e.g., migration/acculturation, culture-specific family values and organization). However, the present practice model also stresses the cross-cultural common ground between and among all groups—both majority and minority cultural and ethnic groups. Montabo (1994) emphasizes the importance of appreciating sameness between groups; the cross-cultural perception of kinship is the "underlying core of our humanity" (p. 2).

Therapeutic relatedness is best explored by examination of psychodynamic technique, practice, and actual case material to illustrate the treatment process and relationship. This text is organized in accord with the treatment process: the *beginning phase* (referral, assessment, engagement, and therapeutic alliance); the *middle phase* (transference, countertransference, the real relationship, resistance, fixation, regression, and defenses); and the *end phase* (working through and termination). In the context of the treatment process, techniques of psychodynamic therapy (active listening, eliciting information and sharing, advice, mirroring, reflection, attunement, interpretation, suggestion, etc.) are defined and illustrated in the case vignettes. The therapeutic relationship is also differentiated and illustrated in the discussions of case material; these include consideration of the therapist as transference object, selfobject, ego ideal, mentor, teacher, and/or real object.

The use of case material is offered to avoid stereotyping of culturally diverse clients and loss of individualized case planning. In order to ensure that generalizations are not made, the case material in this book presents client (and therapist) histories and ethnic and racial heritages in some detail. Cultural roots and cultural ideals may create conflicts and contradictions for individuals, families, and clinicians because of their diverse and multiple contexts, which span languages, preferences, and subjective experiences. Falicov (1998) cites Rosaldo (1989), who coined the concept "cultural borderlands," with overlapping zones of difference and similarity within and between cultures. Thus in a pluralistic society such as ours, the concept of multiculturalism and of each individual's complex multicultural identity (in terms of race, ethnicity, gender, education, socioeconomic status, occupation, etc.) is apt. For purposes of analyzing the treatment process, the cultural equation and encounter between each client and myself as the clinician are highlighted, to clarify issues of fit–misfit and alliance–misalliance in the therapeutic dyad. Understanding the cultural maps and "cultural borderlands" of clients requires paying close attention to what is shared, as well as what needs to be shared. Thus the therapist's use of curiosity, empathic understanding, and sociological imagination is critical in bridging meaningful gaps with clients from other cultures (Falicov, 1998). Demonstrating and imparting these practice principles are major underlying themes of this text. In excerpts from treatment sessions, the interplay of cultural forces with intrapsychic structure, unconscious forces, and family processes is highlighted.

The majority of the case examples are lengthy accounts of the treatment process and treatment relationship. A few shorter case vignettes are used to illustrate essential elements and characteristics of referral, assessment, engagement, and the therapeutic alliance. All cases have been carefully disguised, to preserve confidentiality; some cases represent combinations of several persons and situations. Where these are appropriate, issues of stigma, discrimination, and racism are noted. The same is true for issues of historic and religious heritage; migration experiences; family structure and family rules and roles; issues of trauma; and legal, medical, economic, and psychiatric realities. Discussions of all these issues, and of planned and unplanned therapeutic interventions, will examine how effective efforts to accommodate diversity were (Altman, 1996).

The overall goal of this text is to assist clinicians in how they listen to and finally hear what patients struggle to share. Ideally, the demonstrated communication process will enable therapists in cross-cultural practice to engage an increasingly diverse client population with greater ease and understanding, as well as with empathic, appropriate attention to cultural realities that are too often either ignored or viewed as marginal to psychodynamic theory and practice. Such therapists will be able to "integrate cultural sensitivity at every step in the process of learning how to observe, how to conceptualize, and how to work therapeutically, regardless of theoretical orientation" (Falicov, 1998, p. 276).

JUDITH MISHNE

Acknowledgments

With deep appreciation and regard, I would like to thank a number of people and institutions for their help and support. I am grateful to The Guilford Press, particularly Acquisitions Editor Rochelle Serwator, for her enthusiastic response to this book, and her help along the way. Her support was invaluable and enabled me to realize my goal of presenting individualized multicultural practice in the context of the treatment process and treatment relationship. I was pleased by the thought and care that went into the book jacket, based on Art Director Paul Gordon's concept of diversity and the therapeutic process. Senior Production Editor Laura Specht Patchkofsky put me at ease in the editing and technical aspects of the preparation of the final manuscript. For many years, Richard Lenert at New York University has been my assistant, and is by now an old and dear friend. He typed the first draft of the manuscript in a timely and accurate way.

I have been privileged to have had the opportunity to teach at a number of graduate school programs, namely, the University of Chicago, Columbia University School of Social Work, and Smith College School of Social Work. For the last several decades my supportive academic home has been New York University School of Social Work, a place that supports faculty and encourages research, writing, teaching, and practice. I am deeply indebted to my colleagues and my students at these schools for stimulating my ever-increasing attention to diversity and multiculturalism. My finest teachers, however, have been my patients, who demonstrated resilience, courage, and personal growth, as they gave themselves and me the opportunity to trust and test out how best to work together in the context of a cross-cultural treatment relationship.

Contents

Prologue: The Changing Paradigms in Clinical Practice

This text demonstrates how a psychoanalytic perspective is useful in front-line practice and work with client populations erroneously considered unable to benefit from insight-oriented treatment. Chapter by chapter, I have attempted to integrate appropriate concepts about race, ethnicity, culture, and gender with psychoanalytic theory, and thus to disabuse the reader of prejudiced views about diverse client groups deemed "untreatable" and unreachable via psychological interventions. I hope thereby to demonstrate responsive multicultural therapy, which strives to establish an empathic therapeutic relationship and treatment alliance.

Psychoanalytically oriented clinical practice has been under attack for several decades. Currently, managed care all but mandates crisis intervention and short-term therapy, and this has affected services for clients and training programs for all clinicians in the mental health professions. In the 1970s, short-term individual therapy, family therapy, and group therapy became preferred, and longer-term psychoanalytic treatment was deplored. Since the 1960s, when social

1

work "turned its lens outward and became engaged in the war on poverty, racism, sexism, civil injustice, and other broad social problems, the status of the direct service practitioner declined and the position of the social activist and social planner was elevated" (Strean, 1996, p. 13).

Different theoretical perspectives also gained ascendancy; these included social learning, role, cognitive, ecological, problem-solving, and systems theories. Ecological and ecosystems theories were the common paradigms used in schools of social work in the 1980s. Emphasis next shifted to empirical research and such models as the task-centered approach, to demonstrate practice efficacy. Many psychology programs abandoned psychodynamic theory altogether and fastened onto cognitive-behavioral approaches; many psychiatry departments shifted to a medical/biological model, in which treatment relied on psychopharmacological approaches rather than psychotherapy.

In some discussions of practice with minority clients, questions have been raised about the usefulness of any psychologically based models, which have been considered inappropriate for various reasons (e.g., their supposed reliance on norms determined by white middle-class standards). Concerns have focused on what is seen as psychoanalytic models' labeling, stereotyping, and stigmatizing of the negative behaviors and patterns within minority families, while ignoring adverse environmental conditions (such as discrimination and institutional racism) and strengths within minority families. According to other critiques, psychoanalytic clinicians target areas of change that have been identified by the clinicians and not the clients, and that are viewed from an individual and cultural-deficit perspective (Devore & Schlesinger, 1987; Shannon, 1970; Willie, Kramer, & Brown, 1973).

Nonpsychological explanations and interventions have been recommended by some. These approaches focus on the social structure inequities resulting from resource disparity, racial discrimination, and barriers in organizational and institutional arrangements. Attempts to resolve such issues at the micro (individual) level are viewed as clearly counterproductive, and so macro-level interventions on behalf of minority populations have utilized community development theories that include social activism and social planning. These gained ascendancy in many schools of social work, especially in the 1960s and 1970s. The focus was on large-scale changes (Middleman & Goldberg, 1974) and included such programs as Head Start and Operation Push. Some author/researchers committed to both micro- and macro-level interventions have developed a combined approach, which includes family systems, behavioral, and task-centered models. This approach is seen as focused on the individual-in-the-environment—a "particularly critical requirement for practice with black families, for whom the impact of cultural and other environmental factors [has] often been ignored" (Freeman, 1990b, p. 44).

Building upon Chestang's (1979) seminal work on black identity and biculturalism, Devore and Schlesinger (1987) and others with a generalist perspective have proposed a number of recommendations for an ethnic-sensitive generic model of practice, which includes work with individuals, families, and communities. Such a model includes consideration of group history, individual history, and group identity as manifested in family coping strategies; in the fluidity of roles and extended family closeness; and in specific family ceremonies, language, and customs. Chestang emphasizes "biculturalism" and supports Norton's (1978) definition of this concept:

> The conscious and systematic process of perceiving, understanding and comparing simultaneously the values, attitudes, and behaviors of the larger societal system with those of the client's immediate family and community system. It is the conscious awareness of the cognitive and attitudinal levels of similarities and differences in the two systems. (p. 3)

The need to view current problems at both micro and macro levels underscores the importance of the clinician's sensitivity to community, individual, and familial problems that are the results of societal racism and discrimination, currently and/or in a family's past. Additionally, there must be awareness of inequitable employment, housing and educational opportunities, and of mislabels and stereotypes (e.g., assumptions about blacks in the mental health system). Finally, consideration of ethnic reality as a source of both strength and strain is also viewed as an important part of ethnic-sensitive practice (Freeman, 1990b). This includes balancing biculturalism with assimilation, and noting that important facets of minority family life include both racial stress and supports via group cohesion.

In the search to effect a reconnection and revitalized collaboration between psychoanalytic theory and social work practice theories, Saari (1996) reviews the history of the social work profession and reminds us of the basis of the chasm that developed and still continues. Academics in social work departments, seeking greater acceptance in the university setting, wanted to offer research; they thus

> began to pay allegiance to the tenets of American behaviorism and of the cognitive movement . . . [and] to examine treatment in a scientific manner which raised questions about treatment efficacy as well as about the validity of its theory base. Clinicians positively influenced by the tradition of psychoanalytic theory reacted negatively to these ideas, knowing that these presumably methodologically pure research efforts failed to capture the essence of the treatment process and that generally, behaviorally oriented treatment interventions were conceptualized at such a concrete level as to miss the individuality of the client and complexity of his or her problems. (pp. 405–406)

Saari further notes that because the treatment relationship cannot be measured in empirical and objective terms, it was downplayed as insignificant, especially in academic research circles during the 1970s and 1980s. This stance has since been refuted by many race/ethnicity experts, who emphatically state that the therapeutic relationship is the critical variable in working with people of color (Comas-Díaz, 1988; Comas-Díaz & Jacobsen, 1991; Jenkins, 1990; Jones, 1985; Jordan, 1991; Thompson, 1989).

My personal perspective on these shifting paradigms in clinical practice may be illuminating here. I have been engaged in social work education for many decades and feel most fortunate to have taught in a number of fine schools, where I have been exposed to a rich array of contrasting perspectives. I have benefited from collegial exchanges with seminal thinkers in the profession. I have included many references and citations to the work of former and current colleagues. Many of my colleagues' views have differed from my own, and from each other's; these differences, I believe, have stimulated my own continued learning and searching to learn how to teach students more effectively, and to employ culturally sensitive practice principles to engage an increasingly diverse client population.

In my first academic position at the University of Chicago School of Social Services, I worked with and learned from a wide array of thinkers. These included leaders in the profession known for their diverse perspectives (e.g., the problem-solving process, the task-centered approach, black identity, and biculturalism). While the school worked and revised its curriculum, innovations and modifications in psychoanalysis were occurring downtown at the Chicago Institute for Psychoanalysis. The writings of Kohut (1971, 1977) were being published while I pursued my own advanced psychoanalytic training at the institute. At that point, the newer concepts in psychoanalytic theory and developmental theory began to be included in courses on both practice and theory at the School of Social Services, as well as in the University of Chicago's psychology and psychiatry departments.

Summers from 1975 to 1982 introduced me to another outstanding array of clinicians and educators as I began an 8-year summer stint at the Smith College School for Social Work. Professional meetings and other Smith activities exposed me to creative and prolific analytically oriented thinkers and writers. The psychoanalytic social work approach at Smith was and remains integral to the curriculum there. My practice colleagues at the Columbia University School of Social Work, where I was employed following my stint in Chicago, challenged this psychoanalytic orientation; at Columbia, the curriculum was reliant on other paradigms (namely, the life model and ecosystems theories).

At New York University, my professional home for more than 20 years, I have worked with stimulating and prolific colleagues steeped in both clinical practice and psychodynamic theory. I have been fortunate to have had the opportunity to become versed in qualitative research methodology, as well as to think more deeply about diversity and multiculturalism, ethnically sensitive practice, and the best ways to share this material with students. The present book is a major step in my considerations about multicultural minority practice.

A psychoanalytic perspective has always felt indispensable to me, both in my own direct practice and in teaching clinical practice courses (Mishne, 1982). It aids me in understanding my clients' presenting problems; in conducting an assessment; and in sensitizing me to my patients' fears and anxieties, both in life and in regard to involvement in the treatment process. The writings of self psychologists and intersubjectivity theorists have provided me with insights that have enabled me to empathize more fully with patients and to be attuned to their concerns, as well as my own responses to the unfolding relationship and treatment process. This relationship includes varied forms of transference and countertransference, as well as the real relationship. I believe that lifelong academic and practicum educational experiences have trained my eyes and ears to attend to both a client's inner world and his or her external reality (which includes environmental realities, such as poverty and violence).

I have found that my own attachment to the psychoanalytic perspective has become ever greater as time goes by, because it assists me in engaging an increasingly unfamiliar population of clients from many different cultures and identities. I have been heartened to see my own endorsement of psychodynamic theory supported by clinicians who have decades of immersion in practice and research with clients of color. Chin (1994) posits that the psychodynamic model is very relevant and applicable to clinical work with women of color, and emphasizes refinement of theory to include issues of color and gender. Likewise, psychoanalytic/psychodynamic theory is an integral part of the integrative approach recommended by Comas-Díaz and Greene (1994a). Comas-Díaz and Jacobsen (1991) earlier observed that clients and therapists both consciously and unconsciously acknowledge their feelings and attitudes about their own ethnic/cultural identities and about differences in the therapeutic dyad. Berzoff, Flanagan, and Hertz (1996) believe that any surrender of a psychodynamic perspective does clients a gross injustice, "because a knowledge of psychodynamic focus can illuminate what is going on in any human interaction of communication no matter how brief it is" (p. 3).

I have become increasingly concerned that without this perspective, direct practice and education for practice will become ever more formulaic, despite the need for varied interventions and methods within a multicultural model of practice. Content about diversity, race, cultures, and subcultures is too often presented with generalizations and stereotypes, lumping people together. "One of the dangers of the emphasis in some schools today on teaching about minorities is that we could neglect the likelihood that no individual is typical, but that each will have absorbed or rejected or differently combined various aspects of that which she has been 'carefully taught' " (Sanville, 1996, p. 423).

As I have noted in the Preface, I believe that the newer psychodynamic theories—such as object relations, self psychology, and intersubjectivity—are extending and modifying traditional psychoanalytic theory and offer essential practice principles for working with increasingly diverse and vulnerable populations. These principles include a two-person "experience-near" perspective, which accommodates patients and empowers them to assert themselves and to demonstrate self-determination and choice of goals. In these new models, clients are viewed as partners in the therapeutic endeavor, not as passive/compliant recipients of treatment. Interpretations and explanations are determined by clients and clinicians together, in what Kohut (1984) called a "new correcting emotional experience."

I feel fortunate to have secured my professional home in a school that, unlike many others, has not abandoned the teaching of theories focused on the intrapsychic, the interpersonal, and the intersubjective. I concur with Saari (1996) that many contemporary educators know nothing about current psychoanalytic theory and models; they mistakenly and commonly refer only to drive theory and other classic concepts, which indeed appear at variance with contemporary multicultural perspectives. They have no knowledge of the newer psychoanalytic models, and seemingly of the recent writings of those attempting to demonstrate the usefulness of these concepts in work with diverse populations (Chin, 1994; Comas-Díaz & Greene, 1994a; Falicov, 1998; Perez Foster, 1998b; Perez Foster, Moskowitz, & Javier, 1996; Thompson, 1989, 1996).

I have found myself intrigued by a book chapter by Leon Williams (1990), a faculty member at Boston College. Williams, like me, has questioned ethnicity as the sole basis for practice with minority clients, because "1) . . . it promotes and encourages dangerous ethnic stereotypes . . . 2) it promotes ethnocentric conflict of the 'we' versus 'they' variety" (p. 181). Williams also cited Lum's (2000) observation that ethnic theories give us nothing new and are simply efforts to synthesize previous principles with ethnic principles. The result is that models of practice relative to impoverished populations are incomplete; important issues for these populations, such as powerlessness, oppression, and discrimination, are left to inferences.

Williams (1990) has *not* advocated a psychodynamic perspective, but rather a generalist approach in which a therapist takes on "role sets" to respond to the range of client issues. An example of such a role set includes the roles of reformer, advocate, broker, and mediator in regard to a client's housing problems, problems with health care, or need for financial assistance. By contrast, the role of clinician is appropriate in regard to resocialization and/or developmental socialization. Williams has proposed developing a national agency to train a coalition of workers for this newly emerging poverty field. Altman (1995) has posited a similar set of roles practitioners must assume in public agency practice, but, in contrast to Williams, he has emphasized utilizing the psychoanalytic/psychodynamic perspective.

Like Altman (1995), I believe that a psychoanalytic perspective empowers the generalist poverty worker to work more effectively with our most vulnerable populations—populations needing the skills of the most able and highly trained professionals. (I also believe that this need for trained poverty workers extends beyond the fields of social work; education, law, and medicine also need to focus on training professionals who can effectively engage with and assist impoverished individuals and families.) Case managers cannot act solely as brokers and referral agents, since separating from clients often causes failed referrals. An all-too-common example is the chronic situation in the field of child welfare, where overwhelmed, distraught parents are given endless one-size-fits-all uniform directives and referrals to obtain a myriad of services. Commonly, they cannot and do not follow through to obtain their GED, parent effectiveness training, membership in a Twelve-Step program for substance abuse, and so on (and on). Without strong clinical skills to effect an empathic and accurate assessment and a supportive referral, overwhelmed workers actually can do little to better the lives of parents who are paralyzed with fear or otherwise psychically depleted and enfeebled. Such parents often cannot utilize the menus offered by case managers, which are frequently presented in an adversarial style, with threats of removal of children. These overworked practitioners need manageable caseloads and skilled supervision to help them develop the needed and appropriate sense of "awe for the complexity of psychological life and some appreciation for the unique ways every individual has of mediating between psychological, cultural, racial and biological variables within and outside of the self" (Berzoff et al., 1996, p. 431).

In his 1990 chapter, Williams said that social work had abandoned black impoverished communities and instead turned to private practice and individual psychotherapy. Studies conducted soon afterward suggest otherwise (Abell & McDonnell, 1990; Butler, 1992); they have found a less bleak situation than the one described by Williams. The vast majority of practitioners remain agency-based, and those who develop private practices do so only slowly and on a part-time basis. It also appears that young workers are not fleeing from taxing client populations, but rather from the constraints and problems that besiege social agencies, hospitals, and clinics (which include poor salaries, enormous caseloads, vast amounts of paperwork, little if any supervision or in-service training, bureaucracies resistive to change, etc.). Clearly, salaries and working conditions for professionals require major attention and change if staff members are to be retained in public agency practice.

It was heartening to see that among those admitted to the New York University School of Social Work PhD class in 2001, half were persons of color; most of these were nonclinician administrators and senior staff members engaged in "poverty work" in front-line public agency settings. With a passionate commitment to remaining agency-based and/or even to opening up new clinics, these doctoral students expressed a profound need for advanced psychodynamic clinical training to help them in their treatment of clients and supervision of staff. They also articulated a strong need for more sophisticated clinical skills and a better grasp of theory, which would enable them to develop and execute worthwhile new programs and interventions, as well as to begin doing needed clinical research.

In sum, I hope that this text proves to be useful and instructive for practitioners, students, and their supervisors in a wide range of clinician training programs, and/or for researchers committed to practice-based research. The text describes clinical work with immigrants and clients of color served at public agencies, as well as those who have achieved middle-class economic status and thus are in treatment with a private practitioner. I have attempted to portray a diverse group of clients in a realistic way, offering considerable detail about their histories, the treatment process, and the treatment relationship. My hope is that the book succeeds in demonstrating empathic, culturally responsive psychodynamic clinical work. This requires the demonstration of valuing diversity, a knowledge of diverse cultures and bicultural phenomena, and a capacity for cultural self-assessment.

PART I

Overview of Cross-Cultural Treatment Considerations

CHAPTER ONE

Views from the 1950s to the 1990s

THE EARLY LITERATURE ON RACE AND CULTURE IN CLINICAL PRACTICE

Since the early 1960s (and, in a few cases, even the 1950s), researchers and clinicians have been examining issues of race and culture in the treatment relationship. The major question has been "whether it is possible to cross racial barriers and provide for meaningful interactions between individuals who have for so long occupied opposing positions in our society" (Ho & McDowell, 1973, p. 165). The early studies only yielded conflicting and inconclusive results, as reported by McRoy, Freeman, Logan, and Blackman (1986). Some emphasized the importance of racial similarity between worker and client (Carkhuff & Pierce, 1967; Vontress, 1971), while others suggested approaches to facilitate cross-cultural client–worker relationships, such as sensitizing to racial issues, developing empathy (Beasley, 1972; Kadushin, 1972; Kautz, 1976; Pinderhughes, 1979), evaluating one's own attitudes and behavior, and using culture-specific approaches or models (Bell & Evan, 1981; Garcia, 1979; Stikes, 1972).

Issues related to power and authority were repeatedly identified in cross-cultural relationships between clients and clinicians, as well as between trainees and supervisors. Student clinicians as reported by McRoy and colleagues (1986) identified the following: "lack of understanding of informal sources of support in minority communities, difficulty in communicating with Spanish-speaking clients, misunderstanding of clients' values and upbringing and difficulty working with older clients who have deeply embedded prejudice" (p. 54). Solomon (1983) cited power dilemmas in unmatched supervisor–trainee dyads: Majority supervisors (and therapists) were frequently concerned about being perceived as racist or patronizing, and thus were often rendered unable to handle issues effectively in cross-cultural and/or cross-racial dyads.

Other pioneer clinicians and researchers focused on racial and cultural issues that affected therapists' countertransference. However, only lip service and marginal attention were given to this early literature, and the efforts of the authors—namely, to highlight obstacles caused by bias, racism, and unrecognized unconscious factors, all of which could impair accurate diagnosis and provision of appropriate clinical services—were largely ignored. Norris and Spurlock (1992), in their review of the early literature, noted that Bernard (1953) and other authors (Calnek, 1970; Obendorf, 1954; Rosen & Frank, 1962; Spiegel, 1976) described how various prejudice-related issues were not always addressed or worked through in the course of a training analysis. Bernard concluded:

> If an analyst has insufficiently analyzed his own unconscious material pertaining to his own group membership and those of others, he and his patients may by insufficiently protected from the interference of a variety of positive and negative countertransference reactions stimulated by the ethnic, religious and racial elements that are present in the analytic situation, the patient's personality, and in the specific content of the patient's material. (p. 259)

Thomas (1962) noted that a clinician's intense race consciousness could cause interpretations to be solely related to racial conflicts, and that this would eliminate the possibility of assisting patients to work through basic problems. Fischer (1971), in contrast, asserted that color-blindness or denial of a black patient's color could cause a therapist to ignore or bypass aggressive and sexual fantasies. Goldberg, Myers, and Zeifman (1974) wrote about white therapists' fantasies that the unconscious of a black patient would differ from that of a white patient. Some therapists, regardless of their racial identity, avoided addressing or acknowledging that a patient was black (Calnek, 1970). Spurlock and Cohen (1969) cautioned readers not to ascribe to the myth that individual treatment would be invalid for deprived populations. They believed that we dehumanize such populations by regarding them as homogeneous groups with stereotypic or undeveloped intrapsychic structures. Meers (1970) suggested that the Hollingshead and Redlich (1958) finding that lower-socioeconomic-status populations did not perceive deviant behavior as mental illness "may reflect the ghetto parent's defensive rationalization or denial: that is to say, families are unprepared to acknowledge the reality of mental illness in the absence of therapeutic help" (p. 211).

It was also observed that inappropriate "positive" countertransference responses could interfere with provision of competent clinical care. An example of this noted by early commentators was so-called "white guilt," whereby clinicians affected by the 1960s civil rights movement preferred and sought out only black clients, for whom they leaned over backward. Welcoming their abuse and acceding unrealistically to their demands (Adams, 1970) were actions that benefitted neither clients nor clinicians. "Some black therapists were known to share in this 'white guilt,' when work with disadvantaged blacks stirred guilt about their own success" (Norris & Spurlock, 1992, p. 94).

In the 1970s and early 1980s, there was what McGoldrick, Pearce, and Giordano (1982) described as a "burgeoning literature on work with a few minority groups, notably black . . . and Hispanic" (p. 8). Unfortunately, as McGoldrick and colleagues noted, these groups were too often depicted solely in terms of their minority or "Third World culture" status. The focus on the harmful effects

of poverty, racism, and political disenfranchisement often completely excluded positive aspects of ethnicity, such as coping skills,
traditions, and belief systems. As a result, this literature overlooked
clients' strengths and instead subscribed to a deficit view. This view
has had a powerful effect on assessment, diagnosis, and treatment of
such clients.

Some white clinicians in more recent years have gotten caught
up in a different problem—the "class, not race" myth (Boyd-Franklin,
1989), which denies the impact of color differences in assessment,
diagnosis, and therapy. Mental health professionals must recognize
that there are vast differences between poor white communities and
poor black communities. In addition, blacks at the middle and
higher end of the economic ladder are not free from stigma or racism, and commonly have less access to employment advancement,
lower self-esteem, and/or discrimination.

Additional problems in appropriate assessment have been recognized as due to clinician bias and prejudice, and to lack of familiarity
with different racial and ethnic groups, causing misdiagnosis. For
example, the same symptoms that are generally labeled as due to
emotional or affective disorders among whites are often attributed to
schizophrenia among blacks (Sota, 1990; Spurlock, 1985). Gardner
(1990) stated that even black doctors are not immune to such bias,
because when they don their physicians' white coats and enter the
predominant white world of health and mental health caregivers,
they often don its values too. Clinicians "of color experience a
unique set of resistances, either because of their own experience of
lack of experience with racism, racial and biracial identity development, cultural and bicultural identity, acculturation issues, class or
religion" (Jackson, 1999, p. 28).

Many culture-based symptoms and syndromes are still so unset-
tling and/or bewildering to majority clinicians that they recoil from,
repress, and/or avoid seeing such patient populations. Language barriers (e.g., with Hispanic clients) can further complicate accurate
cross-cultural diagnosis. Teichner, Cadden, and Berry (1981) found
that because Puerto Ricans are underrepresented in the mental
health professions, professionals' lack of knowledge of Puerto Rican

culture is likely to lead to misdiagnosis. Canino (1990) noted that Hispanic women are more often diagnosed as mentally ill than are men, seemingly because of faulty research instruments that omit "male" disorders. Institutional racism can also cause misdiagnosis. This is manifested in inherent assumptions about pathology (which may be erroneously preidentified, of even normalized, as a cultural trait), and about clients' resistances to treatment (which may actually be due to unrecognized fear) (Spurlock, 1985).

THE IMPACT OF MIGRATION

Recently, clinicians have been forced to move beyond an exclusive focus on issues of class, color, ethnic identity, religion, and national or geographic origin in the face of an enormous wave of migration to the United States. According to the U.S. Bureau of the Census, the foreign-born population increased by 46% between 1970 and 1980, and it increased even more dramatically in the 1980s and 1990s (see Chapter 2).

> The newcomers, who are diverse in age, language, country of origin and culture, have been arriving mainly from Asia, the West Indies, Central America, Africa and Eastern Europe. Their immigration status varies and includes refugees, immigrants, undocumented aliens, entrants and parolees. The Immigration and Naturalization Service (INS), the federal agency assigned to carry out immigration law and policy, determines the status of aliens. The different statuses carry different entitlements to services. These newcomers have been seen by service providers in health, mental health, and educational organizations; family and children's services; and the workplace. (Drachman, 1982, p. 68)

These newly arrived populations compel us to consider and examine the impact of the migration experience, as part of a culturally sensitive response to race and ethnicity.

Although the social work profession has been more involved than any other clinical discipline in service to recent immigrant groups, the response even in social work has been somewhat limited. Professionals are struggling to understand not only the cultures of the newcomers, but also their migration experiences and everything that is entailed in the process of adjusting to life in the United States.

Some researchers, like Drachman and Ryan (1991), see migration as a recurring phenomenon, not a temporary historical event with an emerging ad hoc service delivery pattern of programs that both begin and end quickly. These authors, building on the work of writers in the field and studies of migration, offer a framework of stages in the migration process (Cox, 1985; Keller, 1975). The framework highlights three phases: (1) premigration and departure, (2) transit, and (3) resettlement. It is "assumed that age, family composition, socioeconomic, educational and cultural characteristics, occupation, rural or urban backgrounds, belief systems and social supports interact with the migration process and influence the individual or group experience in each stage" (Drachman, 1982, p. 69). Critical variables in the stages of migration involve such factors as social, political, and economic realities in the home country; separation from friends and family; decisions regarding who leaves and who is left behind; experiences of violence and other life-threatening circumstances; refugee camp or detention center stays of long or short duration; issues of cultural clash; reception from, and opportunity structure in, the host country; discrepancies between expectations and reality; and degree of cumulative stress throughout the migration process.

PSYCHOTHERAPY'S FAILURE TO KEEP PACE WITH CULTURAL CHANGE

Whatever small gains have previously been made by majority mental health practitioners in work with African Americans, long-time resident Hispanic populations, and Native Americans seem to have diminished greatly in recent years, possibly in response to the dramatic demographic changes whereby vast numbers of immigrants are arriving from all over the world. According to Perez Foster (1998a, pp. 253–254), "the domain of clinical practice currently faces a crisis of competence and conscience in the treatment of clients whose ethnicity, race, or class renders them members of minority groups in American society . . . the mental health field as a whole has come to the stunning realization that therapeutic services for ethnically diverse groups lack competent effectiveness" (see also Abramovitz & Murray, 1983; Atkinson, 1985; Sue, 1988; Sue & Sue, 1990). Criticisms have highlighted discriminatory practices directed toward minority groups, therapists' lack of knowledge and understanding of the cultural contexts of their ethnic clients' lives, and the unavailability or inaccessibility of services to immigrant populations (Sue, 1988; Sue & Sue, 1990). Despite the fact that a few early psychoanalyst writers (e.g., Meers, 1970; Spurlock & Cohen, 1969) attempted to refute dangerous bias about ethnic minorities' supposed lack of capacity for individual insight-oriented therapy, Olarte and Lenz (1984) have reported the persistence of the view that racial minority and immigrant groups cannot use individual counseling or psychotherapy, because they lack the capacity for insight and have very limited capability for introspection about the meaning of their experiences and the nature of their relationships.

    In addition to pointing out the paucity of services, Perez Foster (1998a) posits that clinicians' cultural countertransference continues to create impasses in the therapeutic work in cross-cultural therapeutic dyads. Such dyads "provide multiple points of potential dissonance for both clients and therapists, who, upon entering their unique interchange, possess often diverse assumptions about the world around them, their own positions in that world, the meaning of emotional distress, and what is most important, whether [each] will be understood by the other" (p. 256). The four principal areas of the clinician's cultural countertransference, as formulated by Perez Foster (1998a, p. 254), are "intersecting pools of cognitive and affect-laden experiences and beliefs that exist at varying levels of consciousness." They include the therapist's "1) [mainstream] American life values; 2) academically informed theoretical beliefs and practice orientation; 3) personally driven idealizations and prejudices toward ethnic groups; and 4) personally driven biases about [his or her] own ethnicity."

The notion of cultural countertransference is a rich and informative formulation, and one that greatly enhances the entire concept of countertransference. This phenomenon, however, is a complex one, and it can be argued that it is not necessarily absent or nondisruptive even when the therapeutic dyad is culturally matched (see, e.g., Calnek, 1970; Gardner, 1990; Norris & Spurlock, 1992). That is, even when cultural/ethnic/racial congruence exists, patient and clinician can still have very disparate views about mainstream American life values, about the nature and direction of the treatment process and therapeutic relationship, and about their own and other ethnic/racial/religious groups. Indeed, for decades I have heard students in class and clinicians in supervision and consultation exclaim that they have a harder time with clients who are similar to themselves (i.e., of the same race or ethnic group) than with clients who are dissimilar. For example, African American students or practitioners self-report about their frequent severity and loss of professional boundaries with African American clients:

> "I'm harsh and impatient with my African American clients. I can get overidentified, or paternalistic, too directive, too demanding and when they fulfill some of the worst stereotypes about blacks, I all but explode. It's 'cause I really care about them that I want higher/better functioning. I also often feel guilty that I've had it easier, coming as I do from a middle-class, loving, well-educated, intact family, where I had every advantage—the best schools, college and university opportunities, music lessons, travel, sports, family ski holidays . . . all the American dream."

Very similar statements have been made by students regarding their work with Irish clients, Italian clients, or clients of Latin American heritage—whenever there is a matched dyad. The variations of individual and familial beliefs, values, and life experiences are so great that they do not melt away in a therapeutic encounter when patient and clinician are of the same racial or ethnic heritage. "There is tremendous cultural diversity within and between blacks in the United States. . . . There is a need for a constant verification of the reality of individual differences within any cultural group" (Boyd-Franklin, 1989, p. 6). The same heterogeneity must be emphasized when one is considering Hispanic, Asian, African, or Eastern European immigrants. Whatever the reader's views on the sources of acknowledged or unacknowledged cultural countertransference and therapeutic impasses, it appears critical that all clinicians exercise self-awareness and insight into the multiple cognitive and affective factors needed to understand and engage diverse populations, and that they examine the myriad of subjective reactions aroused in the process of improving culturally responsive clinical services that can "manage cultural complexity and respond appropriately to dynamic changes in cultural salience" (Pedersen & Ivey, 1993, p. 13). Cultural responsiveness requires an appreciation of the importance of intersubjective experiences, because culture is so intrinsic to subjective experiences" (Perlmutter, 1996, p. 390).

THE NEED FOR EDUCATION AND SELF-EXAMINATION ABOUT CULTURAL ISSUES

Beginning in the late 1980s, academic institutions and training programs for clinicians of all disciplines have included race-related content. Tatum (1992) has reported that such content generates emotional responses in trainees and students that range from guilt and shame to anger and despair. Tatum has taught courses on the psychology of racism and on racial identity development theory, which eventually require consideration of racism, classism, and sexism. She reports that in classrooms or training settings, anxiety and subsequent resistances quickly emerge. She notes the following sources of resistance:

1) Race is considered a taboo topic for discussion, especially in racially mixed settings. 2) Many students, regardless of racial-group membership, have been socialized to think of the United States as a

just society. 3) Many students, particularly white students, initially deny any personal prejudice, recognizing the impact of racism on other people's lives, but failing to acknowledge its impact on their own. (p. 5)

Since the mid-1990s, cultural diversity, cultural competence, and effective cross-cultural practice have become key topics in clinical education. Racial, ethnic, and cultural diversity are stressed in all national accrediting evaluations of graduate programs that train health and mental health practitioners. Despite the explosion of texts examining various facets of race and ethnicity, these topics commonly remain highly charged, disquieting, and avoided. Because mainstream U.S. culture is obsessed both with notions of "the individual" and with "classification," a struggle ensues between a relentless pursuit of racial and ethnic classification, and discomfort with generalizations and stereotyping.

Examining one's prejudice about one's own race or ethnic origin is a disquieting journey of self-discovery. This form of prejudice is commonly repressed and kept at a preconscious or unconscious level. In a few cases, it explodes and is projected onto others in primitive expressions of bigotry—violence or other hate crimes. More commonly, what is generally apparent is the construction of a myriad of belief symptoms based on "lumping," whereby certain groups are assumed to behave in certain ways because of their color, ethnicity, religion, and/or class. An interesting contrast is that whites are never assumed by whites to behave or achieve in certain ways because they are white. This divisive categorization enforces inferiority and maintains a sense of "the other." More recently white privilege has been recognized and written about, though, like all matters pertaining to race, it is also most difficult to discuss freely and openly. In fact, the very concept of race has been recently challenged by "studies that have demonstrated that there is no acceptable genetic base for the concept of race, and that the divisions of the world into black and white is a delusion of civilization" (Perez Foster et al., 1996, pp. xvi–xvii). Although physical differences between people of different racial groups do exist, what in fact is viewed as problematic by scholars of race/ethnicity is the tremendous social significance given to biological differences in skin color, hair texture, and the like. "Race" as a term is one of the most misused, misunderstood, and often dangerous concepts of the modern world. It has been used to justify some of the most appalling injustices and mistreatments of humans by other humans. It is used in this text, however, "because unfortunately the term is in constant common use, and used extensively by well-meaning analysts and advocates, as well as those who use the term in pejorative and negative ways" (Devore & Schlesinger, 1999, p. 28).

Clinicians and student clinicians, like society at large, are hard put to examine these issues frankly. Commonly, a constricted demeanor is maintained; this runs the gamut from proclamations of color-blindness to politically correct statements regarding multiculturalism. Often there is a reflexive disavowal of bias, fear, and secretly held stereotypic/prejudicial thinking. Thus classes and seminars dealing with ethnic/cultural content are frequently stress-filled courses, replete with silence, disavowals, or anger—especially on the part of the white majority, because this group resents feeling pushed into a *mea culpa* position of having to acknowledge bias or submit to consciousness-raising sessions about cultural diversity. Jackson (1999), focusing on the experience of students of color in diversity courses in mental health programs, has observed that the learning process is impeded by resistances related to "character resistances" (i.e., a defensive coping style that impedes the ability to handle anxiety-provoking material), "resistance to content" (which often evokes memories and recall of painful experiences), and "transference resistances" (i.e., responses to teachers that interfere with communication, trust, and the learning process). In her writings, bell hooks (1989; see also Cohan, 1998) recognizes the alienating quality of much of our speech about race and ethnicity, as well as the extent to which we talk *at* each other instead of *with* each other. Words can be, and often are, used as instruments of exclusion, when indeed there is a need for multiracial bilingualism. A goal of the present text is to reach for such bilingualism, as demonstrated by case material.

Increasingly, clinicians engaged in agency practice and private practice are part of cross-cultural therapeutic dyads. Data provided by the American Psychological Association, the National Association of Social Workers, and the American Psychiatric Association indicate that the overwhelming majority of mental health professionals are non-Hispanic whites (Vargas & Willis, 1994). This trend can only continue in response to population shifts and major demographic transitions (elaborated in Chapter 2). In the mental health arena, the overall situation is a bleak and ever-worsening one as the "domain of clinical practice currently faces a crisis of competence and conscious in the treatment of clients whose ethnicity, race, or class renders them members of minority groups in American society" (Perez Foster, 1998a, pp. 253–254). Criticism focuses on therapists' lack of knowledge and understanding of the cultural context of their ethnic client's lives, and, the lack of adequate appropriate services available to immigrant populations (Sue, 1988; Sue & Sue, 1990). The increased diversity of clients can and does stimulate a myriad of negative feelings and attitudes in therapists. These are commonly unspoken, and many are even "forbidden" attitudes; unrecognized, they can and often do create barriers of inordinate proportions, leading to premature termination and high dropout rates among ethnic clients. The most ominous result is therapeutic nihilism.

THE NEED FOR CHANGES IN THE PROVISION OF THERAPY

The clinical labor force must adapt its therapeutic skills and orientations if it is to meet the challenges of treating ethnic minority clients. One such adaptation is for clinicians to make some fundamental changes in their beliefs about what they must do to work more effectively with clients of diverse ethnic/cultural and linguistic backgrounds. Therapists must earn their credibility rapidly (Sue & Zane, 1987); establish mutual trust early in treatment (Jackson, 1983); and distinguish clearly between cultural influences and individual psychopathology, and make modifications (if needed) in their treatment approaches (Rogler, Malgady, Constantino, & Blumenthal, 1987). Similarly, Zayas, Torres, Malcolm, and DesRosios (1996) note that research supports the following as essential to successfully providing ethnically sensitive therapy: (1) recognizing and expressing the existence of cultural differences between the client and the clinician; (2) having a knowledge of the client's culture; (3) distinguishing between culture and pathology in the assessment phase; and (4) modifying treatment as necessary to accommodate the client's culture. Without a willingness to examine and modify their practice theories and techniques, clinicians will only face the above-noted problems of dropout or premature termination of therapy by culturally diverse clients.

Much of the literature on ethnicity and race is descriptive, and the clinical portions of these writings are directive, offering reflections and suggestions regarding implications for therapy, therapeutic approaches, the role of the therapist, therapeutic techniques, and so forth. What appears to be omitted is the actual human exchange in the *process* of diagnosis and treatment. Most critical (and commonly absent in clinical presentations) are the therapist's inner reflections, inferences, attitudes, feelings, questions, and reservations in the ongoing diagnostic and treatment process. Also rarely available are issues of conventional countertransference, cultural countertransference, and the struggle to modulate and manage the affects and anxieties that are inevitable in multicultural psychotherapy. The contributing roles of the clinical setting and of the therapist's own psychology are seldom (if ever) made explicit in the presentation of clinical case examples. A major goal of this text, through the inclusion of these critical phenomena, is to present vivid accounts of the intersubjective field—that is, the human coexperience in the subjective worlds of client and clinician.

Empathic clinical practice with appropriate attention to cultural realities avoids four typical therapeutic errors. The first one is ignoring a cultural focus altogether. The second is color-blindness—that is, overemphasizing similarities, seeing only universal predicaments, and regarding race and culture as only tangential to therapy. By emphasizing universal similarities and minimizing cultural differences, therapists may actually fall into the trap of ethnocentrism, since they will assume the majority view as the standard of health (Falicov, 1983, 1998; Walsh, 1998). At the other extreme is the third typical error—the position that families are more different than alike. This particularist perspective erases the possibility of generalization about the relationship between an individual or family and the larger culture, resulting in a view only of the intrapsychic system and/or the interior of the family as responsible for everything (Falicov, 1998). The final error is an exclusive focus on ethnicity, which over-emphasizes the concept of shared meanings due to ethnicity, and views members of specific groups as more homogeneous than they really are. This position does not take into account the multiple dimensions of collective identities. There is little room for cultural inconsistencies, dilemmas, and contradictions. The exclusively ethnic-focused approach also assumes objectivity in the observer (Falicov, 1998). Another problem with ethnic-focused generalizations is that culture (which is actually erratic and in constant flux and change) is presented as static and stable; this results in rigid categories and stereotyping. Ethnic stereotyping exaggerates differences between therapists and clients.

Falicov (1998) recommends a "combination-plus approach"—namely, a focus on learning as much about specific cultures as possible, together with a "not-knowing" stance (Anderson & Goolishian, 1988, 1992), based upon curiosity and encouraging a dialogue that incorporates the cultural and personal. This approach provides the therapist with the ever-present "double discourse," which is "an ability to see the universal human similarities that unite us beyond color, class, ethnicity and gender, while simultaneously recognizing and respecting culture-specific differences that exist due to color, class, ethnicity and gender" (Falicov, 1998, p. 275). Falicov's approach is one among several conceptions that are being applied to the practice of culturally sensitive psychotherapy in the 2000s. I discuss such conceptions in more detail in Chapter 2.

CHAPTER TWO

Conceptions of Culturally Responsive Clinical Practice for the 2000s

DEMOGRAPHICS IN THE 2000s, AND THEIR IMPLICATIONS

As noted in Chapter 1, population shifts in contemporary American society are creating enormous dilemmas and challenges in providing clinical services and in training clinicians. The United States is the most ethnically diverse nation in history, and this reality is only increasing as immigration is transforming this country's cities and towns. New York City, the nation's largest city, is in the midst of a major demographic transition that will ultimately transform its cultural, economic, and political life, because 56% of the city's residents are either foreign-born individuals themselves or the children of foreign-born parents (Moss, Townsend, & Tobias, 1997). As of 2000, approximately 37.5% of New York City's population is recognized as foreign born. This figure rivals the high point of immigration for New York City in 1910, when 40% of the city's population was foreign born (Moss et al., 1997). Immigration has altered the ethnic and social composition of the city's total population. In 1990 whites constituted 43.4% of the city's population, but this figure dropped to 38.5% in 1996; the percentage of blacks increased slightly, from 25.4% in 1990 to 26.2% in 1996; the proportion of Hispanics rose from 24.5% in 1990 to 26.6% in 1996; and the percentage of Asians grew from 6.7% of the city's population in 1990 to 8.7% in 1996 (Moss et al., 1997). To varying degrees, similar ethnic and racial trends are discernible across the country.

In the early 1980s, when these distinct immigration trends first emerged, McGoldrick and colleagues (1982) stated that these demographic changes were not increasing mainstream Americans' ability to tolerate differences. The traditional view of U.S. society as a "melting pot" was blinding such Americans to the nation's ever-increasing diversity, and the reality that we are not "melting." These authors also noted that all too many clinicians were being trained with hardly a reference made to ethnicity, as clinics were being set up to serve particular ethnic groups without any staff members who spoke the groups' native languages, and foreign psychiatric residents were being trained without any consideration of the major cultural gaps between themselves and their patients. (Unfortunately, this state of affairs still persists in some areas today.)

Beginning in the 1990s, the concepts of the "melting pot" and assimilation have shifted as the assumptions of a linear model of cultural acquisition have been rejected. Increasing emphasis is being given to the "alternation" model, which posits that an individual "is able to gain competence within two cultures without losing his or her cultural identity or having to choose one culture over the other" (LaFromboise, Coleman, & Gerton, 1993), p. 395). The alternation model stresses the individual's acquisition of skills related to bicultural competence. These skills include, for example, knowledge of the beliefs and values of both cultures, cross-cultural communication competence, a repertoire of roles within both cultures, and bicultural efficacy. Biculturally competent ethnic minority people have been found to have better physical and psychological health than their nonbicultural peers (LaFromboise et al., 1993).

Because of their professional ethics, institutional mission, historic commitment, and accreditation mandates, social work programs have been ahead of other clinical disciplines in attempting to integrate the alternation model, biculturalism, and other issues related to issues of race and ethnicity throughout the curriculum and in the training of clinicians as direct service providers. The teaching and course offerings are uneven, however, varying from school to school. The same may be said about graduate departments of psychology. Only in the last few years has psychiatry belatedly begun to focus on recognizing and teaching about how culture and race affect psychiatric problems. Clearly all these efforts, including the belated ones in psychiatric (and general medical) training, are due to increased immigration: Increasing numbers of psychiatric patients in America come from an array of cultures, presenting syndromes and symptoms that have no equivalent in Western psychiatry. It was not until 1994 that the DSM-IV (American Psychiatric Association, 1994) attached a brief appendix providing an outline for cultural formulations and glossary of culture-based syndromes (see Chapter 3 for a fuller discussion). And only a year or so ago, for the first time, the national guidelines for training psychiatry residents specified that they be trained in assessing the impact of culture on their patients' problems.

CURRENT PERSPECTIVES THAT INFORM CROSS-CULTURAL WORK

Much has recently been written about multicultural practice and the need for competence in working with people from whom one is different. As noted above, the United States is a multitextured society—multiracial, multiethnic, multiclass—in an increasingly diverse world. Dean (2000) has noted that early definitions and categorizations of cultural groups suggested that such groups were static and monolithic; thus "multicultural competence" was originally thought to involve learning about the history and shared characteristics of different groups, and using this knowledge to build bridges and to establish rapport and increase understanding of one's diverse client or patient population. The earliest studies and books (Atkinson,

Morten, & Sue, 1979; McGoldrick et al., 1982; Staples, 1978; Sue, 1981a) contained chapters about the beliefs, practices, and characteristics of different ethnic groups.

By contrast, a second, more contemporary view described by Dean (2000) is that culture is individually and socially constructed. Laird (1998) describes culture as "always contextual, emergent, improvisational, transformational and political; above all, it is a matter of linguistics or of language, of discourse" (pp. 28–29). Dean, commenting on this, raises appropriate questions about multicultural competence in the face of continued change. Her position (which I agree with) is that the concept of multicultural competence is "flawed and typically American," based on the metaphor of American "know-how" and consistent with the belief that knowledge brings control and effective work. She recommends a model of multicultural treatment based on an awareness of "lack of competence"; this model stimulates efforts to gain understanding. This second perspective is the *postmodern view* of cross-cultural practice, which highlights the ever-changing and evolving nature of cultural identities posited by Laird and others, who similarly recommend proceeding with a "not-knowing" position (Anderson & Goolishian, 1988, 1992).

A third perspective on cross-cultural clinical work is a *psychoanalytic intersubjective perspective*, in which the clinician's and client's thoughts and feelings become a field of interaction that operates on multiple levels, within which the client and clinician work to establish trust and to construct meaning together. Perez Foster (1999) considers the effects of a therapist's "American" values, academic theories, practice orientations, personal biases, and prejudices about his or her own racial/ethnic identity and those of clients, using a similar psychoanalytic approach. Comas-Díaz and Jacobsen (1991) observe that race, ethnicity, and culture activate deep unconscious feelings and "become matters for projection by both patient and therapist, usually in the form of transference and countertransference" (p. 401). (The intersubjective perspective is discussed in more detail in the next section.)

Dean (2000) considers a fourth perspective, which moves the

lens from the interpersonal to that of a *macro-level sociopolitical perspective* or level of analysis. She notes that Green (1998) considers the dynamic interplay between oppression, prejudice, discrimination, and the lack of economic opportunities on the one hand, and individual and familial characteristics of those suffering endless and systematic oppression on the other.

Dean's (2000) central thesis is the need to work from a basis of evolving understanding that is the outgrowth of an interested and open mind. As clinicians, we must be eager to engage clients, rather than to categorize and/or stereotype them based on our "knowledge" of characteristics of specific racial and/or ethnic groups. We must continually question and revise our views about our clients' behaviors and beliefs. We need to struggle to see and contain experiences of both sameness and differences.

THE INTERSUBJECTIVE PERSPECTIVE AND SELF PSYCHOLOGY

"Intersubjectivity theory," like self psychology, is a psychodynamic theory commonly referred to by clinicians attempting to provide culturally sensitive, empathic, and responsive clinical services. It should be noted that intersubjectivity theory is not considered an outgrowth of self psychology, nor is its intent that of superseding self psychology. According to Stolorow (1994), the two developed in parallel, and intersubjectivity theory was greatly enriched by self psychology's framework. Stolorow perceives the concept of the "intersubjective field," which consists of "the reciprocal interplay between two (or more) subjective worlds," as a theoretical construct "precisely matched to the methodology of empathic introspection" (p. 38). Further comparisons are provided by Trop (1994). He points out that both theories are relational, and that both reject the concept of drive as a primary motivational source. Both theories use empathy and introspection as central guiding principles. However, self psychology is centered on the concepts of selfobject and selfobject transferences; in contrast, the "motivational principle of intersubjectivity theory is not centered in the concept of selfobject, but is more broad based, striving to organize and order experience" (p. 78). Trop also emphasizes the unconscious organization of experience, and posits that intersubjectivity theory is "uniquely suited to facilitate a clinical understanding of the patterning and thematizing of experiences when selfobject functions are missing" (p. 89). In contrast, a self-psychological perspective aims to promote a steady internalization of the therapist's selfobject functions. The goal of the "curative process is the patient's enhanced capacity to choose more mature selfobjects in future relationships" (p. 89).

In an earlier work, Stolorow, Brandchaft, Atwood, and Lachmann (1987) have described transference as an "instance of organizing activity, a microcosm of the patient's total psychological life, and from this perspective it is neither a regression to, or a displacement from the past, but rather, an expression of the continuing influence of organizing principles and imagery that's conceptualized out of the patient's early formative experiences" (p. 36). These authors emphasize the psychological processes of organizing current experiences, to which both patient and therapist contribute. These authors particularly stress the analyst's contribution to the transference and disagree with the traditional view that it originates entirely from the patient. Stolorow and colleagues posit that any action, lack of action, or restricted action or attitude by the clinician affects the transference. Thus they conclude that the "transference and countertransference together form an intersubjective system of reciprocal mutual influence" (p. 42). In this intersubjective approach or two-person psychology, the clinician's actual contribution to the transference must be acknowledged, to give the patient freedom from having to accept the clinician's organizing principles and psychic reality. From this perspective, the patient's view of the therapist is neither debated nor confirmed; rather, perceptions are explored for comprehension of the meanings and organizing principles that define the patient's psychic reality.

Those clinicians whose primary focus is on culturally responsive clinical practice are raising questions, like Stolorow and colleagues, regarding the effectiveness of traditional unicultural psychodynamic training and treatment. Since it only provides guidelines for the patient's exploration of feelings, but omits the therapist's own character and inner life, the traditional one-person perspective is "limited in its capacity to accommodate differences, racial, cultural or socioeconomic, in the psychoanalytic dyad" (Altman, 1996, p. 197). Perez Foster (1996) concurs: "The recognition of the contributing role of the therapist's own psychology in psychodynamically oriented work could not be more vital than in its treatment of patients whose culture, race, or class markedly differs from that of the therapist" (p. 17). Altman (1996) goes on to assert that a two-person treatment model is necessary for taking account of cultural, racial/ethnic, and class differences within the psychoanalysis, and that a three-person perspective is needed for taking account of the clinic or community context in which psychoanalytic work with a culturally diverse clientele often occurs. The two-person perspective focuses attention on the interpersonal intersubjective field between client and clinician, and the three-person model additionally includes the context (e.g., the impact of a public clinic on the treatment work). The one-person perspective with an anonymous clinician does not fit with the conditions of a social agency, hospital, or public clinic, where in fact therapists commonly engage in interracial, intercultural, and interclass therapy work, and where they must often fulfill multiple roles (e.g., as advocates for patients, and as brokers to procure entitlements and/or emergency items such as cash, food, and housing).

OTHER PERSPECTIVES UTILIZED IN CROSS-CULTURAL TREATMENT

In addition to utilizing newer psychoanalytic models to accommodate diversity, culturally sensitive clinicians are using theories and models that are not rooted in psychoanalysis or psychology at all, but rather in sociology, anthropology, linguistics, and other fields. Treatment of diverse populations requires that clinicians be sensitive to sociocultural patterns and to the reality of "cultural relativism."

Fish (1996) states that "sociocultural awareness is quite like the sociological concept of class consciousness, except that it is an awareness relating to membership in virtually any group with similar backgrounds or in similar situations, and not just an economic class" (p. 129).

All of the researchers and writers examining clinical work with culturally diverse individuals emphasize the need for clinicians to be aware of their own cultural identities and their personal attitudes toward and beliefs about other ethnic groups, because these will influence their relationship with patients. Pinderhughes (1982, 1989) recommends self-questioning about one's feelings about belonging to one's culture and ethnic group; one's positive and negative feelings about one's ethnic and cultural identity; and one's experience as a person either having or lacking power in relation to ethnic and cultural identity, class identity, and sexual or professional identity. Until recently, these types of questions were only researched and explored by sociologists and anthropologists. Now psychotherapists are also considering them.

Narrative theory and narratives are also providing clinicians with a framework to assist clients in constructing explanations that promote more adaptive functioning.

> Narrative theory has developed from a convergence of trends in a variety of disciplines. Major theoretical roots rely on developments related to linguistics and language acquisition (Vygotsky, 1978, 1986), symbolic interaction (McCall & Wittner, 1990) and hermeneutics (Packer, 1985). These newer areas of inquiry study the interpretation and structure of experiences. Narratives can tie together events, behaviors, perceptions, affects, and memories, in an attempt to make sense of the world. Narratives continuously are constructed and revised and are used to evaluate the past in light of the present. (Ware & Levy, 1996, p. 404)

Saari (1991) notes that since narratives are part and parcel of treatment and the interpretive process, the role of therapists with their patients is that of co-constructors of meaning. Narratives can serve to enable clients to reflect on their inner lives and their world views, and to share these with their therapists.

An initial major goal in culturally sensitive, optimally responsive treatment is engaging a client and beginning a meaningful collaborative interaction—one in which the client experiences attunement, attentive listening, spontaneity, empathy, and evidence of the therapist's emotional availability. In order to engage and connect, the client needs to experience the therapist's desire to be educated about the client's values, preferences, world view, and belief system. The therapist can often provide help in the client's development, over time, of a coherent narrative. Such a narrative commonly has a central or major organizing theme, which serves to integrate dissimilar experiences into a coherent whole, thereby providing or enhancing a sense of personal meaning, personal continuity, and survival (e.g., in the face of adversity).

In the cross-cultural dyad, the therapist may be challenged with a totally unfamiliar cultural context, which requires being educated and informed by the client about specific rituals, customs, beliefs, and such. This education is often presented by way of shared narratives. Therapists can also be faced with symptoms and syndromes that bewilder and alarm them, because they have never before encountered these. This reality requires setting aside long-held views about pathology and symptomatology, in order to avoid misdiagnosis or premature clinical decisions. Specialists in clinical cultural competence like Dr. Arthur Kleinman, medical anthropologist and psychiatrist at Harvard Medical School, note that there are American psychiatric syndromes unique to Western industrialized societies and not seen elsewhere: "Anorexia nervosa seems as culture-bound to America as amok is to Malaysia" (Kleinman, as quoted in Goleman, 1995).

THE NEED FOR MORE TRAINING
FOR MAJORITY AND MINORITY CLINICIANS

Clinicians, both experienced and inexperienced, need more training and education about how to offer diverse client populations a professional relationship that reflects acceptance, respect, interest, and warmth. The hope is to create what is called a "safe holding environment" in which a trusting exchange can take place. This is a challenging goal in all therapeutic efforts; it becomes more demanding and complex if a majority clinician is inexperienced in working with minority populations, if a clinician is struggling with his or her own racial and ethnic identity, and/or if there must be an intermediary (e.g., a translator) to facilitate the dialogue between client and clinician. Given the racial, ethnic, and cultural diversity of immigrants, and the general homogeneity of mental health providers (who are predominantly white and middle-class), cross-cultural therapeutic dyads often cannot be avoided. Such dyads indeed constitute a fact of life in the mental health field, which has as yet not attracted or recruited sufficient teachers and students from a diverse array of cultures. The existent few minority therapists also need more training and supervision, especially when treating patients from the majority culture. Tang and Gardner (1999) posit that for African American clinicians race exerts great power in the treatment process, whereas for Chinese American clinicians culture is the dominant factor. These authors indicate overlap in the themes of transference to them as members of different racial minorities, based on racial and cultural stereotypes and projections, which are often key to patients' inner lives.

Minority and majority therapists alike can fall prey to overgeneralization, which can "result in cultural reification, harmful stereotyping, and loss of the individuality that is so important in effective treatment and case management. In fact, intracultural differences may exceed intercultural differences in some cases" (Sue, 1981b). All clinicians need to become less positivistic and assertive about human nature, and more willing to shape psychodynamic meaning through reciprocal interactions with clients (Perez Foster, 1998b). The culture and cultural borderlands of clients and therapist provide both with "powerful metaphors and rich resources with which to introduce change possibilities. When this is combined with an appreciation of the intersubjective meanings for both clients and therapist, culturally responsive and effective therapy indeed becomes possible" (Perlmutter, 1996, p. 400).

PART II

The Beginning Phase
of the Treatment Process

CHAPTER THREE

Referral, Assessment, and Diagnosis

SPECIFIC ISSUES IN THE ASSESSMENT AND DIAGNOSIS OF CULTURALLY DIVERSE INDIVIDUALS

An in-depth consideration of culture is essential in the process of assessment, case formulation, and diagnosis of culturally diverse individuals. As clinicians, we should have some knowledge of our patients' cultural identities, but that alone is far from adequate. Immigrants and refugees are arriving from such diverse places, and due to such unfamiliar life events and circumstances, that we must not feel certain about our actual knowledge of clients' histories, cultural values, and customs. Rather, we must offer open minds, warmth, and a manner that conveys our interest and eagerness to learn from our clients. It is also important for us as clinicians to explore the beliefs and affects that inform our views of ourselves and their clients as cultural initiatives (Dean, 2000).

As noted in Chapter 2, the American Psychiatric Association

(1994) has belatedly acknowledged the impact of culture and ethnicity on diagnosis and treatment, as stated in the introduction to DSM-IV:

> Special efforts have been made in the preparation of DSM-IV to incorporate an awareness that the manual is used in culturally diverse populations in the United States and internationally. Clinicians are called upon to evaluate individuals from numerous different ethnic groups and cultural backgrounds (including many who are recent immigrants). Diagnostic assessment can be especially challenging when a clinician from one ethnic or cultural group uses the DSM-IV Classification to evaluate an individual from a different ethnic or cultural group. A clinician who is unfamiliar with the nuances of an individual's cultural frame of reference may incorrectly judge as psychopathology those normal variations in behavior, belief, or experience that are particular to the individual's culture. (p. xxiv)

Lu, Lim, and Mezzich (1995) add: "Aspects of cultural formulation include assessing a patient's cultural identity and understanding how culture affects the explanation of the individual's illness, support system and the clinician–patient relationship, as well as understanding how culture affects the assessment and diagnosis of culturally diverse individuals" (p. 479).

The following items constitute the DSM-IV outline for cultural formulation (American Psychiatric Association, 1994):

Cultural identity of the individual (i.e., ethnic or cultural reference groups; degree of involvement in culture of origin and host culture; and language or languages used and preferred).

Cultural explanations of the individual's illness (e.g., nerves, somatic complaints, possessing spirits).

Cultural factors related to psychosocial environment and levels of functioning (e.g., stress in the local social environment; support provided by religion and kin networks).

Cultural elements of the relationship between the individual and the clinician (e.g., differences in culture and social status; diffi-

culties emerging due to language problems; problems in ne-
gotiating a working relationship).

Overall cultural assessment for diagnosis and care (i.e., all cultural
considerations that influence comprehensive diagnosis and
care).

Finally, in conducting the diagnostic study or assessment of a
young client and family from another culture or another part of the
world, one must be clear about the developmental norms in the culture of origin. What are specific as well as typical parenting patterns
and expectations of age-appropriate tasks? Commonly, there is cultural dissonance when some members in a family acquire a bicultural perspective and others do not. Children and adolescents
often acquire specific American behavior styles and mores; these can
and frequently do put them at great odds with their parents, who often choose to reject American standards and expectations, remaining
attached to parenting practices and expectations from their culture
or country of origin. However, as common as this pattern of genera-
tional conflict is, it is essential not to stereotype recent immigrant
and/or minority families by assuming that it always occurs. Again,
the key to understanding is to learn, as best one can, what indeed is
happening in the family one is working with.

BASIC PRINCIPLES OF PRACTICE
IN THE BEGINNING PHASE

The beginning phase of treatment consists of referral, assessment,
diagnosis, selection of appropriate interventions, and initial engagement, ideally culminating in the development of a working alliance
that is based on the growing treatment relationship between client
and therapist. This chapter discusses the tasks of referral, assessment, and diagnosis; engagement and development of the working
alliance are considered in Chapter 4.

According to Basch (1980), what a clinician does formally in an initial interview is in many ways not much different from what all of us do, intuitively, all the time in other relationships. We continually form impressions of the person to whom we are talking, becoming aware of the feelings stirred up within ourselves, and of the thoughts and memories stimulated by the conversation, all the while we monitor the content of what is being said. "One's final judgment about the interaction is as much based on one's inner reflections as on what the other person has actually said" (Basch, 1980, p. 3). In the same way, when listening as clinicians to our patients, we form some opinion of their characters, what they want with us, and whether or not we feel what they want is reasonable and feasible; we then determine how we will go about communicating and implementing our agreement with, or our rejection of, their implicit and explicit wishes. We listen and attempt to identify various levels of meaning with patients we are seeing for the first time, and to minimize anxiety about this initial encounter, we attempt to become acquainted with the patients. We can learn a great deal by observing how the patients sound (e.g., anxious, guilty, matter-of-fact, oblivious, or condescending), and by examining what feelings the patients stir up in us, the clinicians. As Basch again notes, "It is the therapist's inner reactions that are most important in evaluating a patient's situation, especially if there are discrepancies between the communications the patient is trying to make, and the reactions he arouses" (p. 4).

The psychotherapeutic process is significantly informed by the initial interview, which tends to set the stage and the tone for subsequent sessions. Basch (1980) cautions against "tendentious investigation of the patient's past with a view to explaining his problems by blaming them on what in essence has been visited upon him by life, [reinforcing] the belief, often already present, that he is a 'victim' entitled to compensation and relief" (p. 11). This would result in the clinician's being pushed into the role of rescuer. To learn how a client orders and understands his or her world (or fails to do so) requires that the client not be bombarded with a series of preconceived questions, which would relieve him or her of having to adapt creatively to the session and the therapist. The clinician's immediate task is to become aware of his or her own hunches and impressions, and to avoid coming to premature conclusions about the client and the client's problems. The goal of every initial interview is to allow client and clinician to become acquainted. Some clients may need more support and structure than others in sharing information in a cogent and coherent manner. What is critical is to mobilize each patient to speak about him- or herself; what the patient is avoiding generally becomes obvious, and it can then become the focus for the clinician's eventual comments and further exploration.

Bacal (1998a) refutes the classic concept that the treatment process inherently includes professional detachment and distancing— that is, "optimal frustration" (Bernfeld, 1928; A. Freud, 1946). He has introduced the term "optimal responsiveness" (Bacal, 1985), which refers to the therapist's acts of communicating understanding to the patient. The optimal response tends to evolve out of empathic immersion and empathic intersubjective resonance (i.e., the patient's knowledge that his or her affect has been shared by another).

REFERRAL

The process of a referral, and the therapist's response to the referral, set the tenor and tone both of the assessment and of the treatment process as a whole. In regard to referral of a child client, Kessler (1966) has emphasized that the referral should communicate genuine concern for the child's welfare, rather than portraying the child as a disruptive nuisance. It should emphasize the child's and parents' inner feelings, pain, and confusion, and involve the parents in preliminary work that deals with their initial resistances and objections. The latter are frequently related to fear of stigma or disability, concern about confidentiality, or guilt. Other causes of parents' resistance to a referral enumerated by Kessler include jealousy; rivalry with the therapist; displacement of conflict between the parents onto the therapist; the child's and a parent's sharing the same constellation of defenses and symptoms; the need to fail in accord with masochistic character traits; and/or anxiety about the results, due to fear of the unknown. Many of these issues are also germane in referral of an adolescent and/or adult client.

Some patients (or parents of patients) present an ongoing transference conflict, expressed as resentment of authority, professionals, and experts. Such a conflict may be especially likely when a patient has been referred for treatment by an outside institution or agency (a school, the courts, etc.). The situation is often exacerbated when a client and therapist are of different racial, ethnic, or cultural groups: Cultural countertransference and insufficient sensitivity to a client's values and beliefs may cause the case to conclude abruptly. In this instance the cultural clash produces irreconcilable differences, so that treatment flounders or never actually begins. I believe that all of these factors were evident in the case of Laura, described later in this chapter.

ASSESSMENT AND DIAGNOSIS

During the assessment or the earliest stage of treatment, ideally, the client (for parents) and therapist will come to have the same psychological conception of the problem. A beginning alliance between therapist and client evolves out of assessment activities such as history taking; educational explanations of behavior, normality, symptoms, and defenses; and provision of preliminary advice and recommendations regarding methods of discipline and age-appropriate behavior (for parents), recreational activities, and other issues. All of this is easier said than done.

The process of evaluation and assigning a diagnostic label is not meant as, and should not be perceived by the client as, a pejorative depreciation or stigmatizing effort. A diagnosis, rather, is a shorthand description of the client's presenting problem(s), underlying character structure, and physical state, as well as the nature of his or her milieu and environmental stressors. The diagnosis should offer information about the client's and family's strengths and weaknesses, and thereby provide guidelines for optimal treatment planning. The distinction between evaluation and treatment is not merely a semantic one. A basic confusion is introduced when initial contacts are regarded as treatment, before any insight is gained about the structure, nature, and history of the problems. A client and therapist cannot genuinely engage in mutual goal setting before the client has a better understanding of his or her presenting problems and the reasons why a particular therapeutic modality is being offered. The client needs to comprehend the nature of the prescribed therapy, including an estimate of the time and cost involved. As I have noted elsewhere (Mishne, 1983):

> Beginning treatment before formulating a diagnosis is analogous to prescribing antibiotics indiscriminately for any undiagnosed physical disease. There are various modalities of ongoing intervention, but few agencies and clinics provide the full range. Without a diagnostic assessment, clients may simply be forced into whatever modality a given agency offers, with no differentiation of case need. The reality that an agency cannot be all things to all people and rather should, on appropriate occasions, refer clients elsewhere, underscores the need for assessment as a separate and distinct phase. (p. 27)

Basch (1980) states that most of the disorders treated in clinical practice fall into three groups: the symptom disorders (e.g., the psychoneurotic character disorders), the narcissistic or selfobject disorders, and the borderline disturbances.

> These diagnoses describe vicissitudes of development and cannot be based on the patient's appearances, phenomenology, or presenting complaint. Only an evaluation of the patient's overall character structure, especially as it emerges in his relationship to the therapist, can establish the diagnosis. However, even though a diagnosis carries significant implications for treatment and for prognosis, the categories are not hard and fast or mutually exclusive; they can overlap. Furthermore, the therapist's diagnostic impression can change, either as he comes to know the patient better or as the patient matures in treatment. (p. 105)

In considering what impedes an individual's development and/ or ability to cope, consideration must be given to fixation and regression (see Chapter 7 for a fuller discussion). In a situation of fixation, the clinician notes the tendency in psychic development for residual elements of earlier phases to gain and hold strong "charges" of psychic energy. This causes various degrees of persistence of primitive, often childlike ways of thinking and relating to people. In addition to constitutional reasons for arrest, there may have been early experiences in childhood when the client's developing ego was overwhelmed by stress. Traumatic experiences such as parental loss, lengthy separations from parents, and critical illness usually involve a harmful combination of extreme frustration and extreme gratification (Mishne, 1997). Trauma can also cause regression, for example, libidinal regression manifested by a falling back or retreat to an earlier phase of instinctual organization (e.g., a latency-age child's decompensation and resumption of night fears, separation-anxiety, and thumb-sucking following the death of a parent) or ego regression (manifested by a retreat to an earlier stage of mental organization (such as when an adolescent reverts to infantile, stubborn, or tormenting anal behaviors and ways of thinking of very early childhood). The contrast between arrest and regression indicates that in cases of regression, a higher level of development has been reached and then lost or abandoned.

In assessment of a child patient, Anna Freud (1962) notes that

since neither symptomatology nor life tasks can be taken as reliable guides to the assessment of mental health or illness in childhood, we are left with the alternative idea that capacities for growth are the most significant factors in determining a child's mental health. Accordingly, it becomes the diagnostician's task to ascertain where a given child stands on the developmental scale, whether his position is age-adequate, retarded or precocious and in what respect and to what extent the observable internal and external circumstances and existent symptoms are interfering with the possibilities of future growth. (pp. 149–150)

To determine where a young child or an adolescent stands on the developmental scale, Kessler (1966) has suggested scrutiny of (1) the discrepancy between the child's chronological and behavioral ages; (2) the frequency and character of the symptoms; (3) the number of symptoms; (4) the degree of social disadvantage; (5) the intractability of the behavior; (6) the child's personality or general adjustment; and (7) the degree of the child's inner suffering. These factors inform the clinician of areas of strength and weakness in the child and family, and indicate how and in what respects the child handles age-appropriate tasks, despite his or her symptoms. Such issues also suggest hypotheses about possible contaminating factors, be they past, present, constitutional, or family induced. Simultaneous assessment of the child's parents permits the clinician to ascertain the extent to which they not only contribute to the maintenance of the child's problems, but also support healthy aspects of the child's personality. Assessment of major psychological traumas in the child's parents and other family members is crucial, as is general information about the structure of the family and extended family. The parents' interpersonal relationships, employment, and financial base, values, ethnicity, culture, and lifestyle must also be explored.

In all assessments of children, adolescents, and adults, it is critical to note how information is shared. The importance of this goes far beyond obtaining factual data about illness, separations, and the like. Indeed, the emotional tone in a family, and the attitudes, feelings, and styles of family members' relating, are more telling than mere hard data and facts. The clinician must be alert to affects of depression, anger, anxiety, aloofness, and indifference. Do members of a family present apathy, anger, helplessness, enthusiasm, or empathy? (Mishne, 1997). Issues of motivation, and the voluntary or involuntary nature of help seeking, are commonly key prognostic issues that serve as guidelines for the ongoing planning for therapy.

There is a spectrum of psychotherapy to consider when one is making treatment decisions and recommendations. This includes supportive treatment at one end, and intensive, insight-oriented, uncovering psychotherapy at the other. Supportive therapy is generally aimed at symptom relief and overt behavioral change, without emphasis on changes of personality or resolution of unconscious conflict. The goals of insight-directed treatment are more ambitious; they require that the patient possess a high degree of psychological-mindedness, insight, and intelligence to permit scrutiny of and understanding of his or her own mental processes, whereby the patient is helped to become conscious of previous preconscious or unconscious material.

CASE OF CARLOS: EXAMPLE OF REFERRAL AND ASSESSMENT OF A PUERTO RICAN ADOLESCENT

Carlos was a 14-year-old Puerto Rican boy referred to me for outpatient treatment by his mother, at the suggestion of a social worker who was a friend of the family. He had had several previous outpatient and inpatient treatments because of two serious suicide attempts. At the time of the referral to me, Carlos had run away at midnight from the hospital and was hiding out at the home of an adult friend, maintaining phone contact with his mother, but refusing to come home unless she promised he could stay at home and not be returned to the hospital.

The hospital reports described Carlos as angry and defensive, not working in therapy, and showing no gains in insight or self-control. He evidenced no motivation for treatment, but the reports recommended that he continue to be treated in a long-term, closed, and secure setting. The unit director at the hospital (a state institution) felt helpless in the face of recent policy conflicts between the hospital and the fire department. He described the fire department's prohibition of locked windows, which had resulted in several adolescent patients' running away at night, when staff coverage was lighter than during the day. Because of prevailing conditions at the hospital, he recommended that outpatient work be attempted, if Carlos's mother could control his activities and school attendance. Given her history of difficulty in handling Carlos, however, the prognosis appeared guarded.

Carlos's behavior problems dated back to the fourth grade, when he was frequently truant from school. He was identified as becoming depressed at the onset of puberty, 2 years before his first hospitalization. The depression markedly intensified 1 year before the outpatient assessment, when he made his first suicide attempt by taking three-fourths of a bottle of antibiotics, following a fight with his girl-friend. Initially, he was referred to and seen in a special outpatient child depression clinic. The staff there felt he responded positively to the medication (imipramine in dosages up to 225 mg/day) and noted a decrease in depression and irritability. However, Carlos was dis-charged from the clinic after 5 months because of poor compliance and failure to keep appointments.

Carlos's mother and her common-law husband, who lived with the family, described Carlos as being very changeable in mood. One day he would be sweet and gentle; the next day he would have a dev-ilish look on his face and seem to be looking for trouble. They said he was erratic in his exchanges both with them and with his younger brother. He could get into violent fights with his brother, destroying his toys and punching him very hard. Both adults were fearful that he would really hurt his brother.

Carlos's second suicide attempt followed an argument with his mother over his late hours. He had arrived home very late and fought when his mother attempted to admonish and reason with him. In the course of the argument, he threw a fire extinguisher against the wall of the kitchen. When the argument subsided and the adults went to bed, Carlos wrote several suicide notes to his family and close friends, went into the bathroom, and took twenty or thirty 325-mg Tylenol tablets. He reported going to bed hoping to "wake up dead," clearly a denial of the reality that he could destroy himself. He awoke early the next morning and phoned a nurse at the depres-sion clinic where he had been treated the year before. She phoned an ambulance, which took him to the hospital emergency room, where he was treated with syrup of ipecac and Mucomyst. His hospital emergency room care was uncomplicated, but he required constant supervision, as he was assessed by the psychiatric consultant as a suicide risk. Therefore, with parental consent, he was then trans-ferred to a psychiatric inpatient setting.

At the time of this first inpatient admission, Carlos was dressed in black and was wearing two live rifle bullets, according to the case records. He showed a preoccupation with suicidal ideation, and a fascination with death, violence, and violent crimes. He spoke of identifying with the character played by Charles Bronson in the movie *Death Wish*. He described his mood as "sad." His affect appeared constricted, and he was guarded and made little eye contact during the interview. There was paucity of speech, and he was hesitant and spoke in a soft voice, though at a normal rate. There was no evidence of psychomotor agitation or retardation, bizarre thoughts, delusions, or hallucinations; memory appeared intact. Suicidal ideation was admitted. Judgment and insight were poor, and Carlos did not believe he needed hospitalization or any treatment. He was admitted as an involuntary patient.

Carlos came from a working-class Puerto Rican family. He was the older of his mother's two sons (fathered by different men). His brother was 3 years younger and was described as more communicative and less moody and erratic than Carlos. The mother was a most attractive small woman, who was clearly bewildered, frightened, and overwhelmed by her son. She acknowledged delegating too much responsibility to Carlos when he was younger, and having a non-parental (sometimes sibling-like and sometimes quasi-marital) relationship with him in the immediate past, considering him the man of the household. Until recently, the mother had had sole financial responsibility for herself and her boys, and had frequently been overwhelmed by struggling to maintain employment and provide her children with adequate care and supervision. She had relied on her mother, sister, and relatives in Puerto Rico to care for them. There had been separations and a variety of residences for the boys and their mother in the past.

At the time of the first hospital admission interview, the mother's lover of several years was residing with the family, awaiting his divorce; he and the mother planned to marry. This man appeared to be a strong, secure, stable, and caring father figure. However, he was deeply resented by Carlos, who felt his authority in the home had been usurped. Carlos defied him and his mother, stayed out late, associated with rough, acting-out children, and was frequently truant from school. Presumably he was not involved with drugs or actual crime, though the mother and her common-law husband feared this in the future, given his current peer affiliations, history of petty shoplifting, and contacts with street gangs. At the time his outpatient therapy with me began, following his elopement from the second hospital, he was obsessively preoccupied with a brigade of youths committed to subway safety. He wore Army camouflage fatigues, boots, and a beret, and carried a nightstick. With elaborate grandiosity, he proclaimed that he was a brigadier general in his organization.

During the course of his first hospitalization, Carlos's behavior had ranged from pleasant to cooperative to hostile and sarcastic. He did not appear depressed, sad, or given to tears (these affects had been noted at home). He demonstrated good ability to relate to adults and peers, and exhibited humor and warmth toward the other adolescents. Continued preoccupations with violence and violent crimes dominated his interests, however; he clipped endless articles about crimes of violence against women, or crimes involving dismemberment and mutilation committed by teenagers against their parents. All of these, he stated, should be controlled by the police and adolescent gangs "warring for peace and order." When angry, he would make verbal threats of violence to peers and hospital staff, but he did not act out aggressively, as he did at home and on the streets of his neighborhood.

After some opposition to the evaluation process in the hospital, Carlos was formally tested by the psychologist, on two separate occasions. His intellectual functioning was rated in the low average (87) range on a Verbal IQ scale, but in the very superior range (133) on a Performance IQ scale, with an average Full Scale IQ of 110. The enormous discrepancy between the Verbal and Performance scores seemed to be due to his unusual manual and visual–motor skills and his failure to acquire age-appropriate academic skills and knowledge. His general knowledge and his reading and arithmetic skills were particularly poor. This action-oriented rather than verbal means of problem solving stimulated impulsivity, since it was coupled with an inability to think through and anticipate the consequences of his actions. No signs of psychotic thinking were evident. Reality testing was unimpaired. Grandiosity was noted; Carlos could not tolerate having his depression viewed as rooted in his sense of rejection and deprivation. His mother was this adolescent's lifeline, and his attempts to separate from her and accept his "stepfather" were thought to be causing his current decompensation.

During the course of Carlos's first hospitalization, he remained angry and defensive and did not work in therapy. Thus he showed no gains in insight or motivation for continued therapy. Long-term hospitalization was recommended because of his need for a closed, protected setting; at the conclusion of the family's limited insurance coverage, he was transferred to a well-staffed long-term adolescent unit in a state hospital. He was opposed to continued care and threatened legal action to get himself discharged. He presented himself as a victim of other people's ideas. In the second hospital, he showed no evidence of psychosis and no delusions; he presented a full range of affects and related directly with a good amount of eye contact. Nevertheless, his history of suicidal, impulsive behavior, and his noncompliance with inpatient and outpatient therapy and reasonable parental limits, suggested his continued need for a safe, closed, structured setting.

In both hospitals, and later as an outpatient, Carlos described a repeated experience of seeing a lady dressed in a white veil standing in his room, as he was about to fall asleep. He descried her as "my admirer," as "she is ready to marry me." He said he believed that the apparition was really there and was not a hallucination. He claimed not to be afraid of it, as he believed it to be his guardian angel. Also, he claimed to experience hearing his name called sometimes by a relative or a friend, but when he went to the door, no one was there.

These hallucination-like experiences appeared to be linked to his mother—his guardian angel—and his mother's Hispanic absorption in witchcraft, spells, curses, devils, and the like. Carlos, emotionally unseparated from her, shared her spiritual system and her concerns and preoccupations with feeling haunted. With great fear, the mother described to me how she placed charms over doorways and elsewhere, and she shared her fears with what she claimed was complete openness for the first time. The mother said that she was sharing with me what she'd never spoken about before, because she trusted me and believed that I really cared about her and her son. In particular, she feared a curse from her lover's legal wife (this divorce, as noted above, was not yet final). She linked her son's crying and sleep disturbances with her own similar symptoms. The mother described how Carlos became obsessed with devils (drawing devil faces) and ideas of death as possibly related to her fear of the devil and his wish to "rescue" her. He often dressed in black and claimed he had to stalk the cemetery and confront the devil.

The outpatient treatment with me could not be sustained, because Carlos's old behavior problems erupted and escalated after his first week at home. He kept late hours, despite the adults' rules and requests; he was truant from school; and he fought with other students in the playground, resulting in school suspensions and nocturnal wandering. Carlos quickly became erratic or very tardy in attending therapy sessions. He seemed afraid of (though also relieved at) sharing thoughts, images, and fantasies in sessions, in the context of a growing degree of rapport and attachment to me as the therapist. After 1 month at home, Carlos regressed to sleeping on the floor, crying, and throwing temper tantrums. He articulated grandiose, toddler-like fantasies of superhuman techniques of survival (e.g., how he could live even if he tied his hands and ankles, weighted himself with stones, and leaped off a high bridge into a river).

His "stepfather" and mother, in agreement with my recommendations, became convinced of the necessity for rehospitalization. The "stepfather" was quick and responsive, whereas the mother seemed more confused, apprehensive, and fearful of her son's hatred of her if she signed him in, even though she acknowledged that she could not protect or limit him at home. Carlos's rehospitalization proceeded smoothly. His mother described with amazement her son's actual relief at the adults' decision to accept my recommendation that he required a closed and protective setting.

Rebellious and acting-out behaviors are not uncommon for the adolescent junior high school population. However, assessment distinguishes between what is "age-appropriate" deviation and symptoms that are grossly interfering with a child's progressive line of development. The DSM-IV models suggest an Axis I diagnosis of oppositional defiant disorder (313.81) as an appropriate clinical diagnosis; additionally, cyclothymic disorder (301.13) must be provisionally noted, given Carlos's hypomanic symptoms and numerous periods with depressive symptoms and suicidal ideation. Axis II, which specifies personality disorder, suggests borderline pathology due to Carlos's failure to separate and individuate from the mother, such that in their "open" system he shares her anxieties and magical thinking. This borderline diagnosis corresponds to a developmental perspective, reflecting Carlos's immaturity and lack of more adequate age-appropriate functioning.

DISCUSSION OF ETHNIC/CULTURAL ISSUES IN THE REFERRAL AND ASSESSMENT OF CARLOS AND BRIEF TREATMENT OF HIS MOTHER

Carlos was seen in an extended diagnostic evaluation offered on a crisis basis, since he was at risk, having left the hospital against medical advice. His lack of separation/individuation seemed apparent in his sharing his mother's self-described Hispanic immersion in witchcraft, spells, curses, devils, and the like. Carlos was not assessed as psychotic, but rather as a highly suggestible, nonfunctioning adolescent with low-level borderline disturbance, in urgent need of rehospitalization. He was too agitated and acting out to truly connect and make any sort of relationship with professionals, inpatient or outpatient.

Carlos's mother was provided with crisis-interventive supportive psychotherapy, and she did respond positively to me as her clinician. She was able to reveal information never before shared with any health care provider, because she felt a special rapport with me and a sense of trust in my efforts to help her and her son. She was appreciative of being seen immediately, on a scaled low-fee basis, by the "former professor" of the friend who had referred her. She had been provided with this information, and so the typical anonymity was absent in our relationship. The mother was able to talk about the "forbidden topics" of spells, witchcraft, curses, and the like, as well as her sense of fear and guilt at being involved with a man who was not yet free and divorced, which she believed warranted punishment and retaliation from her lover's still-legal wife.

Although I utilized a psychoanalytic perspective in my work with Carlos and his mother, I concur with Roland's (1996) caution about the need for a new paradigm, which includes psychological phenomena that psychoanalysis regards with suspicion:

> Patients from a variety of cultures are involved in this world in a number of ways, related to, for example, astrology, palmistry, the spirit world, psychics, mediums and rituals. This is an anathema to most psychoanalysts. Psychoanalysts coming from a tradition of the self-contained, rational individual simply do not appreciate that patients outside of the Northern European/North American culture will have a self that is not only far more enmeshed and embedded in an extended family/group/community context . . . but often also in a world of invisible influences. To assume a denigrating attitude towards these psychological phenomena will be to miss a major portion of these patient's psyches. (p. 88)

Had I not been able to accept the mother's attachment to the world of spirits, which was so important to her, I would have missed understanding her and would not have been able to form and sustain a professional helping relationship with her.

Carlos's mother also spoke about the sense of fear and vulnerability that seemed pervasive in her immigrant family. Not only was the mother having problems with Carlos, but her sister and her sister's son were concurrently suffering from trauma, due to the murder of a friend of her sister. Because I was able to secure an immediate referral for the mother's sister and nephew in the nearby state where they resided, the mother felt a familial sense of being protected in the context of our professional relationship. She articulated her gratitude for my help, and perceived my acceptance of her ethnic and cultural belief system and values, as well as her customs and rituals.

She continually felt the need to thank me with presents—for instance, home-cooked Puerto Rican specialties, and (when I was departing for a vacation) a number of beach-towel-like sarongs for my holiday at the beach. Under other circumstances I do not and would not want to accept presents from clients, but in this case I believed that rejecting this woman's offerings, as well as attempting to engage her in analyzing her need to bestow gifts, was contraindicated. I felt that her cultural customs required my graciously accepting her offerings, and I was comfortable and willing to alter and modify more classic therapy practices and techniques, in keeping with her needs. I also was willing to assume an active advocacy role in regard both to seeking help for her sister and nephew, and to securing a rehospitalization plan for Carlos.

This overwrought mother was able to vividly share her ethnic reality, as well as her struggles with racism and prior poverty (due to unemployment, underemployment, and frequent unscrupulous underpayment). She had gone back and forth between New York City and Puerto Rico, but was not able to function with bicultural ease. Despite proficiency with spoken English, she had been stymied repeatedly in attempts to enroll in classes to improve her reading and writing in English, and thereby to improve her skills and compete more effectively in the workforce.

Over and beyond the crisis with Carlos, the mother was able to trust me enough to share her concerns about herself and the reasons for her sense of powerlessness. Because this woman could share her historic background and current struggles regarding immigration, family, and general adaptation to her two communities (here and in Puerto Rico), we were able to work well together in a relationship that evidenced warmth, rapport, trust, and openness. I admired her courage and felt great compassion and respect for her. We kept in touch, via follow-up, in regard to Carlos's rehospitalization and subsequent referral to and placement in a residential treatment center. The mother also accepted a referral for herself to secure long-term therapy and parent guidance, at an agency specializing in work with Hispanic families and staffed with an atypical number of Spanish-speaking social workers.

CASE OF LAURA: EXAMPLE OF REFERRAL
AND ASSESSMENT OF A BIRACIAL
PRESCHOOLER AND HER PARENTS

Laura's mother, Ms. B, was referred to me for help for her daughter by a friend and work colleague who had had a long and close relationship with me. Laura, age 3½, was enrolled in a nursery program whose staff members were raising questions about their ability to manage her because of her repeated aggressive outbursts. In fact, at the time of the referral, Laura was being maintained at her nursery with one staff person assigned to closely supervise and contain her, with the proviso that the parents secure professional help as soon as possible; if they did not follow through, Laura would be excluded from school. Ms. B and her husband thereby felt angry and resentful at being forced to seek the services of a child therapist, and arrived with a "chip on their shoulders."

Mr. and Ms. B were an upper-middle-class, highly paid interracial couple, working in television advertising. The father, an attractive and well-educated black man, was more than 15 years older than his wife. He was openly resentful that he had acceded to his wife's desire to have a child, since he had two grown children from a prior marriage. He felt too old to be dealing with a preschooler, and acknowledged that Laura was a handful both at home and at school. The mother acknowledged the same, but also indicated enjoying Laura, though she often felt frustrated at how hard Laura was to handle (especially when it came to limits, bedtime, and the like). Despite this acknowledgment of their own stresses in parenting Laura, both parents felt that the school was excessively demanding in their expectations of Laura.

What was most striking was Mr. and Ms. B's steadfast commitment to continuing their style of child rearing, which was most unusual. Namely, the mother still persisted in nursing Laura; both parents bathed with Laura; and at times both parents were quite punitive in spanking her—a practice employed daily, concurrent with endless overindulgence of her regarding food, late-night hours, TV watching, and endless purchases of anything and everything she might mention or ask for.

I was asked to contact the nursery school and its director, and the staff indicated feeling very overwhelmed by Laura and her parents. Laura, a large child for her age, was described as barely containable and frankly somewhat frightening to peers and staff alike. When she'd explode, she could throw a tricycle across the room at a child who might have angered her. The parents were described by the school staff as argumentative and uncooperative.

I found myself troubled that I also experienced Mr. and Ms. B as argumentative and uncooperative, and pondered whether I was possibly struggling with some latent sense of bias about the racial intermarriage (O'Neal, Brown, & Abadie, 1997), and/or with any negative cultural countertransference feelings toward Mr. B. To the best of my ability, I explored my experiences and feelings about interracial couples and African American males. In my own friendship circles, I have had ties over the years with two interracial couples; I have also had meaningful friendships with a number of African Americans, including several African American males I met in college, in graduate school, and over the years as colleagues at various places of employment.

What I did find most troublesome was the shared resistance by Mr. and Ms. B to contemplating any questions or self-doubts about their parenting practices. The mother seemed to have no questions about nursing this very large, articulate child, in my office and/or wherever Laura would demand to be fed. Likewise, the father had no questions about his admitted practice of rather severe nightly spankings, when his patience would run out as Laura resisted going to bed at 10:00, 11:00, or 12:00 P.M. Because I was feeling the school's pressures to expel Laura (a reality the parents seemingly refused to see), I realize retrospectively that I attempted to move in too quickly with parent guidance and advice. My aim was to attempt to help the parents handle their daughter in a more age-appropriate fashion and with greater limits, boundaries, and consistencies, empathically expressed. I was unsuccessful in effecting any changes, and I now believe this was because I moved in too quickly, minus a relationship of rapport and trust. In retrospect, I feel that I was responding only to what I considered to be Laura's needs, as well as the needs of her teachers, and did not allow sufficient time to embrace the parents' needs as well. I wanted to try to stave off Laura's expulsion from her school.

Any and all advice about weaning Laura and curtailing the spankings was met with fierce parental resistance. The mother informed me that she had no interest in her pediatrician's or my advice, or the advice rendered in all books she'd read about parenting, about ending the nursing process. Since Laura and she supposedly enjoyed the nursing, and since the mother knew that at her and her husband's ages, there'd be no more babies, she intended to continue to nurse for as long as possible. The father was equally adamant about his continued reliance on spanking, and presented his decisions and feelings with a racial and anti-Semitic edge (e.g., "No Jewish white middle-class advice is worth a damn. Don't you know that we blacks spank our kids and believe in this as best?").

I was unsuccessful in trying to show the parents the consequences of excessive overgratification, overstimulation with shared baths and showers, and excessive frustration stemming from spankings (all of which I feared were becoming eroticized). I was equally unsuccessful in helping the parents contemplate the link between their aggressiveness and Laura's, which she'd displace onto teachers and peers in her acting out at school. Because there was no diminution of Laura's outbursts at school, or in her parents' outbursts in parent–teacher conferences, Laura was expelled as had been threatened. The parents' anger at the school expanded to include me, for not having convinced the school to keep their child, and for not magically producing another program that was ready and willing to admit Laura. When the parents concluded their contact with me, Laura was only provisionally enrolled at a public school Head Start program; the program staff demanded that the mother also attend, to contain her daughter. The parents rationalized all these events as due to racism and bias about their interracial marriage and their interracial child. They had no grasp of the realities of Laura's emotional problems and interpersonal dilemmas.

With such a young child, any diagnostic label is tentative and provisional. The DSM-IV model of assessment would suggest a diagnosis of oppositional defiant disorder (313.81), whereas a developmental perspective would suggest Laura's borderline pathology due to a failure to separate/individuate from her mother (who for her own needs—even possible borderline pathology—held onto Laura via the inappropriate nursing, etc.). Pine (1974) might perceive Laura as a child "on the way" to borderline pathology.

DISCUSSION OF ETHNIC/CULTURAL ISSUES IN THE REFERRAL AND ASSESSMENT OF LAURA AND HER PARENTS

As noted earlier, I have pondered my atypical and striking lack of success with this case. It would be easy to write it off as "one of those impossible cases that no one could work with successfully." Although it was true that the parents were in a locked-horns struggle with their daughter's school, was it inevitable that the same had to occur in treatment? I have more questions than answers about this case, and cannot readily say that the outcome was inevitable. Despite decades of experience in practice, I realize that the bulk of my cases have been voluntary, self-referred, motivated clients, eagerly seeking help for themselves and/or their children. I acknowledge less comfort in clinical work with nonvoluntary, resistant patients engaged in self-injurious and/or excessively aggressive interchanges with their spouses/partners and/or their children. I knew that this case could not appropriately be reported to child welfare services, in that the spankings administered would not be viewed as child abuse, but rather as parental discipline (they were severe, but not severe enough to result in documentable physical injury to Laura). Moreover, I knew that such an action would further inflame and/or enrage the parents, who would take out their frustrations on their child, thereby worsening the situation.

At no time during the referral and the assessment were the parents receptive to my view of their problems with Laura. We did not share the same psychological conception of the problem, and were not able to begin to form an alliance (which commonly occurs during the assessment activities of history taking and educational explanations of a child's behavior, when I attempt to offer preliminary advice and recommendations about methods of discipline and age-appropriate behaviors). The parents saw the school's insistent referral as one that portrayed both their child and themselves as disruptive nuisances. In retrospect, I believe that I was put off by the parents' anger and sense of being persecuted. I did not attempt to engage in routine information gathering about their respective backgrounds and marriage, due to my sense of urgency about staving off Laura's threatened expulsion. My not learning about their world view was also due to my sensing the father's scorn and anti-Semitism. Lerner (1992) has noted that "confronting Black anti-Semitism is particularly difficult for liberal and progressive Jews" (p. 125). Because progressive Jews are used to viewing blacks as innocent victims of racism, it can be hard to accept them as being guilty of bigotry (Langman, 1999). Gates (1994) states that "attention to Black anti-Semitism is crucial, however discomforting, in no small part because the moral credibility of our struggle against racism hangs in the balance" (pp. 217–218).

Although not attacking defenses is appropriate (particularly early in the assessment process), I believe retrospectively that I was atypically avoidant in confronting the racial issues in this case, out of a conviction that the father's projection of his own racism might be too hot to handle. I did not adequately explore their parting accusation of racism on the part of the nursery school (and possibly, implicitly, on my part, as well), out of a sense of frustration at not having been able to connect with and engage this couple. I have had decades of successful cross-racial work with African American clients, and have enjoyed some meaningful lifelong friendships with African Americans; I felt insulted at being misperceived by this couple as a white Jewish professional with strains of bigotry.

I have pondered whether my own sense of injury and racial countertransference contributed to the parents' premature termination and departure from ongoing therapeutic contact. I had not had the opportunity or made the time to attempt to explore the themes of racism, prejudice, and discrimination that Mr. and Ms. B had possibly endured from the dominant society. I had assumed that this would be revealed eventually in our ongoing contact. Because of their affluent socioeconomic status and high educational level, I had possibly erred in assuming that they were adept and sophisticated in dealing with whatever racism they encountered. My fear of paternalism and/or of any sense of patronizing them was possibly based on my own particular sample of African American friends and colleagues, who are quite adept in dealing with racism-related issues. I may have erred by stereotyping Mr. and Ms. B in accord with the socioeconomic and educational attainments of other black and/or interracial couples I have known. If I had the opportunity to work with Mr. and Ms. B again, I would not succumb to the pressures from a child's school to such an extent that I failed to consider the ethnicity and culture of an interracial couple early in the assessment process. I do in fact believe that aside from the difficulties "inherent in any congenial bond, interracial couples must deal with the reality that their differing races or ethnicities create problems of their own" (Davidson, 1992, cited in O'Neal et al., 1997, p. 28). I confess that I probably would be less cautious with an interethnic couple than with an interracial couple in exploring the life history and marital relationship. My reflexive response was reinforced by Mr. and Ms. B's overt anger, and by their ego-syntonic comfort with child-rearing practices so at variance with my own views and values. I recognized some strains of helplessness behind the parental spankings, but also realized belatedly that I was struggling with my own feelings about their narcissistic use of Laura—their doing with her what suited them (i.e., the nursing and shared bathing). In addition, I was put off by the uniquely negative response this couple elicited from me, due to the aforementioned issues. In retrospect, I do not think I gave this unpleasant reaction and its possible causes enough thoughtful self-scrutiny to understand them. I rationalized away my own feelings, "reassuring" myself that Mr. and Ms. B had similar problems with the staff at their child's school.

With the leisure of hindsight, I have come to reaccept and recognize the clinical reality that no one can expect to be successful with all cases. Given these parents' general level of hostility toward their child's school, as well as their child, anyone would have been hard put to effect change and/or gains quickly. Again, however, I do believe I moved too quickly to attempt to alter their dysfunctional parenting patterns, out of my hope to stave off Laura's expulsion from her school. I believe that the parents could not tolerate this rejection from the school, and that following it they would have then rejected any and all therapeutic efforts as well. In reviewing this case for this book, I was and remain impressed with the staying power of feelings of failure in clinical work with occasional cases. As clinicians, we can intellectually understand and explain a negative therapeutic response; nevertheless, the stress of unsuccessful cases commonly remains unaltered or relieved by time.

CHAPTER FOUR

Engagement and Therapeutic Alliance

The engagement process and the establishment of a relationship between clinician and client have been preoccupations of the helping professions for decades (see, e.g., Robinson, 1930). It is well recognized that people will be more open and free with those who they trust to "hold their confidences, to pay attention to their story, to accept and to understand them. The professional relationship has certain features that distinguish it from personal and other lay relationships; from the practitioner's point of view, it is always client-focused" (Meyer, 1993, p. 45).

Interviewing is an art. In part, it consists of skills that can be improved and eventually perfected, primarily through continual practice. Garrett (1972) points out, however, that practice alone is not enough. In addition, communication in a professional conversation must convey tact; careful, attentive listening; empathy; and recognition of both the conscious and unconscious aspects of human motivation. In seeking to help people even in very simple situations, we need to listen not only to their explicit comments and requests, but also to the undertones that reveal their feelings and give us clues to perhaps even more serious (and not overtly revealed) situations (Garrett, 1972).

CASE OF SARAH: EXAMPLE OF ENGAGEMENT WITH AN AFRICAN AMERICAN WOMAN

When Sarah called initially to request an appointment for a consultation, she explained that she was fairly new in the city, having moved from the Midwest, where she'd completed graduate school. She had been referred by a therapist she worked with intensively during the summer between the first and second years of her master's degree program, when she'd gotten quite depressed and ambivalent about finishing her degree. She said she was feeling uncertain and depressed again, and was ready to engage in therapy to deal with this recurrent problem, once and for all. We agreed on a time to meet and scheduled our first appointment. In discussing the location and address of my office, Sarah said lightly, in a breezy way, that she was familiar with the location of my office and the upper west side of New York City, because of where she resided. She gave me her address and offhandedly stated that her apartment was actually in Harlem. Neither of us missed a beat, or said any more on the phone about this. But it was my distinct impression that Sarah felt she needed to forewarn me that she was black.

She arrived punctually, a very tall, slender, attractive, and articulate African American woman, 34 years of age. During the first half of our initial session, she referred to her need to mention Harlem, and it was as I'd suspected. Because we were meeting for the first time, she felt the need to alert me to the fact that she was a person of color, hoping that I would not have a problem about this and that it would not be a barrier to my working with her, if she felt comfortable with and wanted to work with me. Her presentation of her racial identity, originally oblique and understated, then became a major focus in the engagement process. Sarah asked whether I was experienced in working with clients of color, and was quite specific in raising questions and in seeking information. In turn, I was open and disclosed quite a bit about my professional training and experience. Contrary to classic technique and emphasis on anonymity, or turning the question back to the patient as an issue to explore, I was very open with Sarah about my cross-cultural and cross-racial experiences with both patients and colleagues of color. I frankly informed Sarah that, in fact, the vast majority of my cross-racial professional experiences have been with African Americans—adults, children/adolescents, and their parents—and that I have also had substantial experience in working with Hispanic clients (and, by contrast, very minimal contact with or experience with Asian patients). Just as clients in general have a right to ask about therapists' training and orientation, I believe that clients of color have the right to ask white therapists about their actual experiences with racial minority clients.

Because Sarah and I both had resided in the same Midwest city, we also spent quite a bit of time discussing that city and its atypical racial housing patterns in some sections of town. Specifically, once Sarah learned of my prior faculty appointment at the University of Chicago and 10-year residence in Hyde Park, a community famous for its racial integration and harmonious neighborly relationships, she smiled and sat back in relief. She felt calmed and satisfied that I must have had contact with educated professional blacks, and thus maybe even had black friends, just as Sarah had white friends. Therefore, she correctly assumed that hers would not be my first therapy experience with a black professional as the patient.

DISCUSSION OF ETHNIC/CULTURAL/RACIAL ISSUES IN THE ENGAGEMENT WITH SARAH

An important part of the engagement process is beginning where the patient is, and then sensitively helping the patient to become involved in the treatment process. The patient must be reassured that the therapist will attempt to clarify the problems, but that the patient will make decisions and be in charge of his or her life and therapy.

The interviewing process is the vehicle of exploration, and the client is usually the direct source of information. Sarah's focus on both her and my racial identity in the initial interview was understandable, I believe, since she was embarking on an ambitious treatment program. Sarah evidenced a willingness to commit substantial time and money to getting the help she felt would be essential to enable her to be freer, more spontaneous, and better able to make needed changes in her life. Racial identity was a core issue not only in her personal life, but in her professional life—where she perceived institutional racism, but experienced fear, paralysis, and a limited ability to better protect herself. I believe that my willingness to address Sarah's concerns about our different racial identities, and to describe my background in working with clients of different races and ethnicities, played a pivotal role in securing her commitment to the treatment.

THE THERAPEUTIC ALLIANCE

The terms "working alliance" and "therapeutic alliance" have been borrowed from the field of adult psychoanalysis. Discussion of the therapeutic alliance dates from Zetzel's (1956) paper on transference; Greenson's (1965) later paper suggested the term "working alliance." Curtis (1977/1980) noted that in the years from 1950 to 1977, analysts expanded their sphere of interest beyond the patient's intrapsychic life to embrace all aspects of the therapeutic relationship. The therapeutic alliance is not an end unto itself, but rather a means to the end, a way of facilitating the treatment process. It is based upon a new and correct relationship—a "fund of trust" (Basch, 1980, p. 133), in which the patient views the therapist as someone important and skilled with whom he or she is willing to work. In addition to the emerging positive feelings for the therapist, the alliance is based upon the ego's accurate appraisal of a need for understanding and its gratification in being understood. Patients will only look to therapy for relief if they have the capacity for self-observation and some awareness that they have internal problems.

Less well-endowed individuals, with significant ego deficits, often do not "suffer" or experience their symptoms as painful. This is true of some clients with character disorders, who project blame or experience their self-injurious behavior as ego-syntonic. Thus it is apparent that the alliance cannot be taken for granted. "Effective therapy requires a collaborative working relationship in which both partners act on the basis of the implicit confidence in the values and efficacy of persuasion rather than coercion, ideas rather than force, mutuality rather than authoritarian control" (Herman, 1992, p. 136). There are predictable difficulties in forming a therapeutic alliance if a patient has suffered severe traumas, especially in the context of family relationships, which can distort and destroy a capacity for trust.

Basch (1980) has similarly noted that clinicians cannot prove themselves or convince patients of their good will or ability by simple reassurances. Only time and experience together will reassure patients. The development of a therapeutic alliance often proceeds in a tenuous fashion, especially in a cross-racial or cross-cultural therapeutic dyad. The alliance is commonly precarious and fragile, in part because alienation is so prevalent in society today. Meissner (1985) stated that alienation can be viewed as basically a pathology of the self, but one that represents an interface between intrapsychic dynamics and existent social and cultural realities. Alienation includes a basic sense of loneliness and estrangement—continued frustration and chronic despair; combined hopelessness and helplessness. Racism is often a major factor in the alienation experienced by a person of color.

CASE OF SARAH, CONTINUED: EXAMPLE OF THERAPEUTIC ALLIANCE WITH AN AFRICAN AMERICAN WOMAN

Sarah committed herself to an open-ended course of treatment to deal with her long-standing sense of alienation and depression, dating back to the sudden and unexpected death of her mother during her college years. Following her graduation from college and from her master's degree program, she returned home and attempted to reside with her aloof and detached father. This joint residence proved to be too painful, and so Sarah left home, receiving support from one close married cousin, who included her in all family gatherings and holiday celebrations. Despite this link, Sarah basically felt estranged and quite alone, with no larger reference group of black professional peers and no a genuine friendship circle of black peers. Although she clearly self-identified as an African American, her history of peer relations was most atypical for a black woman conscious of her racial identity, in that most of her close friends were white. This dated back to her attendance at an elite private high school, and continued as she progressed through a white-dominated college and graduate school. Her site of employment was also predominantly white—and in her view a tough place to be, given her perception of its covert and long-standing racism, despite the agency's mandate to create and develop low-income and middle-income housing for minority populations. She struggled with her satisfaction with her actual job, as well as with the indignities she endured from her harsh and critical supervisor. She suffered from a sense of insecurity and powerlessness on the job, alongside the knowledge that she was respected by many (if not her supervisor) for her abilities, over and above her position as a "token black" executive.

When Sarah related examples of extremely unpleasant interchanges with her supervisor, she recreated the charged atmosphere at her office, and her pain and waves of self-doubt about her abilities were palpable and painful to witness. I found myself struggling to contain both my reactions of rage at such injustice, and waves of maternal protectiveness for this vulnerable and talented young person, devoid of a parental support system. I have had extensive experience with young adults subjected to extraordinary maltreatment in their workplaces (law firms, academic settings, advertising agencies, arts organizations, etc.), where they must contend with overbearing supervisors, deadlines, impossible demands, long hours, and irrational prima donna antics by people in power. Sarah's situation, although not unique, was distinctly more abusive than any other I've heard of in my decades of contact with young professionals like her. The general level of tolerance for such well-known bullying in an organization can be mind-boggling and extraordinary; in some settings, the harassment may be financial or sexual. In Sarah's work situation, demeaning attacks, outbursts, and foul language were exhibited to many young workers, but toward Sarah, racism seemed to be an additional lethal component. Sarah's workplace lacked the support systems of many organizations, in that there was no office or department of human resources. The sole source of "support" provided to Sarah at the workplace was the option to change her assignment and move to another department in the organization; if she did this, however, she would have to give up handling the tasks that most appealed to her at this job. Ambivalence and indecision characterized Sarah's tenuous handling of this chronic major stressor in her life. Her fears of being fired were exacerbated by the reality that she had no parental support either economically or emotionally, and thereby would have to survive alone, as she was very much on her own. I did not ascribe Sarah's accounts of what transpired at her office as due to her misperceptions or her emotional problems.

DISCUSSION OF ETHNIC/CULTURAL/RACIAL ISSUES IN THE ALLIANCE WITH SARAH

A beginning alliance was apparent in Sarah's commitment to therapy, which arose out of her desire to overcome the emotional inhibitions and difficulties that complicated both her personal and professional life. In this early alliance, Sarah demonstrated a willingness to extend to me "provisional credibility"—that is, a belief that I could help (Basch, 1980, p. 67). I assume that Sarah viewed me as secure in my white racial identity development, whereby I had already achieved an integration of my "sense of Whiteness with a regard for racial/ethnic minorities, . . . and had integrated rational analysis on the one hand, and moral principles on the other, as they relate to a variety of racial/ethnic issues" (Rowe, Bennett, & Atkinson, 1994, p. 141).

Although Sarah had moved all her life in a biracial world, her

African American identity had been shaped by cultural and familial factors, socioeconomic and educational variables, and experiences with racism. When she began treatment, she was quite isolated. She lacked strong kinship bonds, as described earlier; she had close ties with only a very small number of relatives—and, significantly, few to none with her father (who was described as aloof, totally unresponsive, taciturn, and silent, and as having almost completely abandoned her). She was a young, articulate adult of exceptional intelligence and psychological-mindedness, who, despite her many positive attributes, suffered from a sense of insecurity and sense of helplessness. I was certain that her feelings of isolation were not due to her educational and professional attainments or to any sense of guilt at having "made it," since her closest relatives were similarly well-educated successful professionals. Because of her lack of close ties with black peers, I suspected that she had had minimal experiences through early socialization that would have led to a stronger sense of confident black identity. I suspected that the protective setting in her private, predominantly white high school had not prepared her for the racism she subsequently experienced at college, graduate school, and her place of employment. I further suspected that this vulnerability was exacerbated by her loss of her parents—the death of her mother, and her father's subsequent estrangement following his being widowed and depressed. (As our alliance deepened, Sarah told me of her father's long-unresolved marital struggles with her mother. Sarah stated that she believed she reminded her father of her mother, and thereby he displaced his hostility toward her mother onto her.) Although the parental loss and other personal and familial factors figured prominently in Sarah's presenting problems, the issues related to racism in the workplace and her less than confident racial identity appeared to be very significant elements for consideration and therapeutic focus in the work that lay ahead.

Unquestionably, my affirmation of the contextual reality of racism in Sarah's workplace increased the intensity of the treatment alliance (Robinson, 1989) and gave her the motivation to further empower herself (Gutierrez, 1990). At this writing, she has followed my recommendations for pursuing additional graduate work, and in preparation is now taking a course in calculus. Obtaining an MBA will afford her more actual power in the job market than her existent master's degree in public policy does. After 2 years of productive work in treatment, based on an ever-deepening therapeutic alliance, Sarah has been successful in becoming more appropriately self-assertive and self-protective. Most significantly, she has been able to change jobs and negotiate with greater skill and a sense of self-worth regarding her improved salary, title, and responsibilities. She has also made more friendships and social contacts, via her volunteer work (tutoring adolescents, serving as a museum docent) and via forming a book club.

PART III

The Middle Phase
of the Treatment Process

CHAPTER FIVE

The Treatment Relationship

Transference, Countertransference, and the Real Relationship

The middle phase of the treatment process follows the referral, assessment, diagnosis, engagement, and contracting, and may be considered "treatment proper." The deepening relationship between client and therapist commonly reveals transference and countertransference phenomena, as both parties struggle with resistances, drives and drive derivation, ego defenses, superego demands, and conscious and preconscious conflict.

The strategy of supportive treatment involves limited goals and direct relief of symptoms by focusing on the patient's current conscious conflicts and supporting and strengthening defensive and adaptive ego functions to attempt to reestablish an adaptive equilibrium and coping capacities. Underlying unconscious issues and conflicts are not significantly altered. By contrast, insight-oriented therapy aims (to whatever degree possible) to resolve the patient's unconscious conflicts and to promote more effective personality organization and development toward maturity. Symptom relief is secondary, and follows the efforts to resolve underlying conflict.

In this chapter's discussion of the treatment relationship in therapy with culturally diverse clients, the emphasis is on insight-oriented treatment, utilizing newer analytic paradigms, namely, self psychology and intersubjectivity theory. These include the use of empathy and warmth, rather than traditional therapeutic neutrality; a continual emphasis on the interaction between client and therapist in the relationship; and immersion in and sensitivity to the client's cultural context. Both transference and countertransference phenomena are discussed, as is the real relationship between therapist and client.

TRANSFERENCE

Overview of Transference Proper as Manifested by Adult Clients

Although transference and countertransference are psychoanalytic phenomena that generally do not appear in full form in other types of psychotherapy, nonanalyst therapists need to have a clear understanding of them. "There are difficulties in defining these terms, as they often have been misused as catch-all concepts that encompass everything experienced and expressed between patient and therapist. The multiplicity of meanings must be further refined to delineate features pertinent to child patients in contrast to adult patients" (Mishne, 1983, p. 264). In his early considerations of transference, Freud (1912/1958, 1915/1958) stated that all people unconsciously displace and transfer the libidinal aspects of their primary object relationships to their current object relationships. The term "transference," derived from adult psychoanalytic therapy, refers to the patient's views of and relations with significant early childhood objects (parents, siblings, and significant caretakers), as these are expressed in the patient's current perceptions, thoughts, fantasies, feelings, attitudes, and behavior in regard to the analyst (Sandler, Kennedy, & Tyson, 1980). The examination of feelings associated with the patients' prior relationships, and the working through of conflicts associated with these relationships as manifested in the transference, become the bases for modifying and changing maladaptive relationships and behavior patterns.

Self Psychology: Archaic Selfobject Transference

Self psychology posits different transference phenomena for patients with structural deficits who suffer from faulty self-esteem and who are incapable of making clear self–other distinctions. They develop "narcissistic transference" (Kohut, 1971) or "selfobject transference," which must be distinguished from the classic definition and understanding of transference. Selfobject transference phenomena are not the displacement phenomena of classic transference; rather, they involve a use of the therapist to provide a missing part of the self for the client.

There are two main types of selfobject transference: "idealizing transference" and "mirroring transference." The idealizing transference evolves out of insufficiently responded-to early needs for merger with a parental figure who provides strength and calm. In the treatment relationship, the therapist is experienced as all-wise, perfect, and all-powerful (Elson, 1986; Lynch, 1991). Mirroring transferences are divided into three subtypes, related to the patient's level of narcissistic development (Kohut, 1971):

1. "Merger-mirroring transference" is reflective of the most primitive narcissistic pathology, whereby the therapist is experienced as part of the patient's grandiose self and is conceived of only as an extension of the patient. The need for total control of the treatment and the sense of entitlement create rage if and when the patient feels thwarted. Such a patient is taxing and draining, and requires the utmost empathy and restraint on the part of the clinician.

2. The "alter-ego twinship transference" is reflective of greater maturity. There is less archaic emergence of the grandiose self, a greater degree of separateness between patient and clinician, and a better ability to demonstrate partnering and working together. Often

this patient, in search for the perfect twin, has endless disappointing relationships; in treatment, he or she optimally works through this impossible seeking of another with identical views and feelings.

3. "Mirroring transference in the narrower sense" is the most mature form of mirroring transference, with the therapist recognized as separate. In this form of transference, admiration and praise are sought for the patient's narcissistic gratification. When these are unrecognized or withheld, the treatment can be jeopardized.

Kohut recognized that a clinician's reality-oriented remark can constitute a significant rebuff. Statements such as "I'm not an idealized, good, and healthy version of you" led to stalemates in treatment (1978, p. 55). According to classic theory, patients' idealizations are screens or reaction formations against hostile impulses, and they should be so interpreted. By contrast, Kohut proposed that clinicians show greater tolerance of idealizations and deidealizations, as well as the various mirrorings. Empathically delineating and working through mirroring and idealizing transference phenomena can facilitate the reconstruction of the role and function of the archaic selfobjects who failed, in varying degrees, in structure building in infancy and childhood. Treatment aims to stimulate incremental transformation of self and object images, via a process Kohut called "transmuting internalization." Goals center on a development of a healthier and more cohesive self, as the treatment process compensates for failure of empathic responsiveness from parents.

Modifications of Transference in Work with Children and Adolescents

In the course of work with children and adolescents, the relationship is "often a complicated mixture of elements of a real relationship and the extension into the analogies of current relationships and a repetition or even a revival of the past" (Tyson, 1978, p. 213). In 1966, at a panel considering problems of transference with young patients, there was overall consensus that transference neurosis cannot take place in children until there has been sufficient structural development to allow for internalized intersystemic conflicts. Tyson (1978) did not believe that this structural development can be present until the superego becomes independent of parental influence, which usually occurs at the time of puberty or early adolescence. Blos (1972) dated it later; in his view, the infantile neurosis only acquires delineation and structure as a central unconscious conflict in late adolescence, with the greater solidification of the personality. Anna Freud (1971) underscored the reality that the type of personality development and structure that results in an infantile neurosis represents a positive sign of substantial growth. This sort of relatively well-endowed and highly developed child is a rare patient in contemporary clinics and social agencies. More commonly treated are children assessed as "less than neurotic," connoting early traumatic and developmental failures with pre-Oedipal levels of arrest. Due to constitutional deficits, lack of suitable objects, and improper environmental handling, children in this latter group have inferior object relationships; weak identification; incomplete structuralization; permeable id–ego boundaries; and distorted, deformed, and immature egos (A. Freud, 1971).

Tolpin (1978) emphasized that "for patients with structural deficits, genetic reconstructions and interpretations of conflict are ineffectual because these interpretations bypass and obscure the central pathology" (p. 181). Such young patients have faulty self-esteem; lack a sense of direction; and manifest anxiety, depression, and an absence of firm values and ideals. Applying self-psychological concepts to understanding transference phenomena in young patients, Tolpin noted that children diagnosed with disorders of the self develop selfobject transferences, especially merger-mirroring transferences (described earlier).

Because children and adolescents commonly still reside with their parents (i.e., their significant early objects), they generally do not displace feelings, defenses, and perceptions of their past onto their therapists. Rather, more generally they demonstrate the first two of the following four subtypes of transference, identified in Sandler and colleagues (1980); the third and fourth are rarer in juveniles.

1. Habitual modes of relating (i.e., revealing in treatment various aspects of character and behavior, as a child or adolescent would to any person).
2. Transference of the current relationship (i.e., a mode of relating in treatment that is an extension of, or defensive displacement from, the relationship with the primary objects).
3. Transference predominantly of past experience (i.e., the revival of past experiences, conflicts, defenses, and wishes in treatment as a consequence of analytic work, and the displacement of these onto the therapist in the manifest or latent preconscious content).
4. Transference neurosis (i.e., the concentration of the conflicts, repressed infantile wishes, fantasies, etc., on the person of the therapist, together with a relative lessening of their manifestations elsewhere).

Furman (1980) discussed various forms of "externalization" (i.e., attributing any aspect of the self to the external world) in transference. Children and adolescents (as well as "less than neurotic" parents—e.g., those with borderline and other personality disorders) commonly do battle with their environments and use their therapists to represent parts of their personality structure. During adolescent upheaval and rebellion, externalization and projections are common defenses whereby a teenager wards off inner conflict; the superego function is relegated to outside authority figures whom the teenager defies, but also invites to control or punish the displayed disobedience and defiance.

> However, the externalization not only changes an inner battle into an outer one; it also supplants a very harsh inner threat into a usually milder punishment from outside. The visible misbehavior is seen as less of a violation than the inner forbidden activity, or wish, e.g., masturbatory activity or sexual or aggressive feelings towards forbidden objects. (Furman, 1980, p. 271)

The reawakened Oedipal passions often create a profound need for punishment and parental disapproval. If parents and educators either mistakenly fulfill the assigned superego role of harsh disapproval or punishment, or lower their expectations and offer overgratification and permissiveness, they fail to keep the young person in the age-appropriate inner conflict and developmental struggle. Massive frustration and restrictions, overgratification, or an inconsistent and lethal combination of both can create a fertile ground for pathological outcomes. These commonly stimulate the adolescent's regressive sadomasochistic strivings for even harsher punishments and/or failure to develop self-control (Mishne, 1986).

Several specific types of transference phenomena may be associated with a child's or adolescent's habitual style of relating, or with an extension of the relationships with the primary objects (the first two subtypes of transference described by Sandler et al., 1980; see above). Commonly, these patterns (which commonly include various externalizations and projections) will disrupt the therapeutic alliance and obstruct ego growth. Thus they require early identification and active management. Meeks (1971) noted the following problematic adolescent transference phenomena: (1) the erotic transference; (2) the omnipotent transference; (3) the negative transference; and (4) the superego transference (the therapist as superego).

In sum, transference as manifested by most adolescents and children must not be understood to represent displacement from early objects. Children and teenagers residing with parents most commonly evidence thoughts, feelings, and behavior patterns that relate to parents in the here-and-now. Thus there may be nothing special or unique in the way a younger client relates to a clinician; instead, there may be a spillover of current relationships in therapy (Mishne, 1986; Sandler et al., 1980). With a borderline adult client, who is still "residing" emotionally with the maternal object and still unseparated and unindividuated, similar themes and phenomena may occur.

The Intersubjective View of Transference

Just as child therapists caution that transference should not be understood solely as representing displacement from early objects, so too do intersubjectivity therapists raise cautions about, and propose new models and formulations of, transference. They do not concur with the traditional views of transference as regression, displacement, projection, and distortion. Rather, they define transference at the most general level of abstraction, as an instance of organizing activity—an "expression of universal psychological striving to organize experience and construct meanings. The organization of the transference can 1) fulfill cherished hopes and urgent desires; 2) provide moral restraint and self-punishment; 3) aid adaptation to difficult realities; 4) maintain or restore precarious disintegration, prone self and object images; and 5) defensively ward off configurations of experiences that are felt to be conflictual or dangerous" (Stolorow, Brandchaft, Atwood, & Lachmann, 1987, pp. 37–38).

Traditionally, too, transference was understood as emanating entirely from the patient. Intersubjectivity theory challenges that classic position and emphasizes, rather, how the clinician's attitudes and responses affect the transference. Transference and counter-transference are viewed as forming an "intersubjectivity system of reciprocal mutual influence" (Stolorow, Brandchaft, Atwood, & Lachmann, 1987, p. 42). The informed therapist is expected to recognize and acknowledge his or her actual contributions; thus older notions of neutrality and abstinence from action are rejected, in favor of a more active, therapeutic stance of empathic inquiry and demonstrated warmth. Intersubjectivity technique relies on no debate or confirmation of a patient's perspective; instead, the approach is to use the patient's perceptions or points of departure to further explore meaning and the motivating or organizing principles that determine the patient's psychic reality.

Ethnic/Cultural/Racial Transference Phenomena

"For [clients] of color, culture and minority group status set a context of difference that is not 'normal' and expectable in the client–therapist dyad. Projections about race and culture, therefore, will be prominent as transference themes and must be factored in as normal reality issues" (Chin, 1994, p. 207). All patients have feelings and perceptions about their therapists that are influenced by the therapists' authority status. Chin (1994) has introduced the concept of "hierarchical transference" to define this phenomenon. Women of color are described as offering deference to both authority and male figures. When relationships are defined in hierarchical terms, the therapist is commonly perceived as an omniscient advice giver, or as a figure of wisdom and authority whose recommendations must be followed. This hierarchical emphasis can on occasion inhibit spontaneity, but should not be viewed as a communication failure.

"Racial transference" often centers on hierarchial issues (i.e., therapist power vs. client powerlessness and helplessness), especially when a client of color is in treatment with a white therapist. Although power-related disparities and lack of fit, and the resulting perceptions and projections on the client's part, can and do occur in a white matched dyad (e.g., an upper-class social worker from Main Line Philadelphia and an impoverished and uneducated client from Appalachia), the potential for these is commonly far greater in an unmatched dyad of a white clinician and a client of color. Chin (1994) notes that this potential is particularly great when a woman of color is being seen by a white male therapist, since both race- and gender-related factors are at work: Women of color are described as offering deference to both white authority and male figures. The dynamics of racial transference are complex, however, and it can assume different forms when clients of color are in treatment with clinicians of their own race and culture. Although rapport and a positive experience can ensue in matched racial minority dyads, they do not automatically or universally occur. Some clients of color will experience such matched dyads negatively by devaluing the authority and competence of their nonwhite clinicians. Ambivalence and fears of engulfment may also ensue (Comas-Díaz & Jacobsen, 1991).

Chin (1994) also notes that the newer self-psychological concepts of transference (particularly selfobject mirroring transferences) are particularly useful and potent, if expanded and reconceptualized to include empowering and valuing of clients of color, and to support and validate ethnic and gender identity. The newer concepts emphasize empathy between client and therapist, and the importance of the clients feeling understood, via a merger with the therapist in a primitive, infantile, emphatic bond, and identification with the therapist (Kohut, 1977).

In considering transference issues for a diverse client population, one must not focus exclusively on matters of color (e.g., racially matched vs. unmatched dyads), but must consider such characteristics of ethnic groups as a common culture, religion, physical features, language, or some combination of these (Marger, 1997). Other authors emphasize a feeling of affinity (Blauner, 1992): To inhabit a comfort zone, members of an ethnic group congregate together. Gordon (1988) emphasizes a common historic ancestry and identity, which may be coextensive with a particular nation or subpopulation within a nation. Some commentators debate the significance of ethnicity, especially for members of white ethnic groups. Others believe that the nature of ethnic reality is transformed but retained, and still other writers stress ethnicity as giving value and meaning to the lives of group members.

Devore and Schlesinger (1999) emphasize that all ethnic groups in a given society or nation do not have equal status; issues of dominance and hierarchy are everywhere. Thus the transference themes seen among clients of color are also evident in clinical work with members of various ethnic groups, who are responding both consciously and unconsciously to hierarchy, power–powerlessness, oppression, and scapegoating. Cultural transference and cultural countertransference can abound in ethnically unmatched dyads. Ethnic conflict and social stratification or inequality exert profound influence on the lifestyles and life chances of clients and clinicians alike. This includes more affluent, more highly educated minority groups, which are considered "middle-man minorities" (Marger, 1997), vulnerable to scapegoating and hostility from those at both the top and the bottom of the prestige hierarchy. In the United States, the clearest examples of "middle-man minorities" are Jewish and Asian people. These are relevant facts in clinical practice, given the high proportion of Jewish clinicians.

Traditional psychosocial/psychodynamic clinical practice has been criticized for not offering a "clear and detailed indication of how minority status, ethnicity and class converge to shape individuals and contributes to the problems for which they seek help. A second omission is the tendency to stress the negative and dysfunctional aspects of the ethnic reality. The unique and often beneficial effects of membership in various groups [are] often ignored, and/or bypassed" (Devore & Schlesinger, 1999, p. 117). Other critiques note that attention to ethnic reality is not incorporated routinely and sensitively into interventive procedures, or that while attention is given to ethnicity, socioeconomic status is not adequately incorporated.

Hierarchical issues of power–submission and other aspects of cultural transference are very much affected by style, language, and nonverbal communication. How people communicate cross-culturally is crucial. "Western values often stress getting one's point across, for example, whereas Asian values stress politeness in verbal discourse. As a result, Westerners tend to value verbal fluency, while Asians tend to value listening and not interrupting others" (Chin, 1994, p. 210). Language and linguistic modes often convey significant semantic differences in the therapeutic relationship. Chin (1994) notes that several writers (DeLaCancela, 1985; Marcos & Urcuyo, 1979) have described how bilingual Latina clients will switch between languages in psychotherapy to express difficult emotional experiences and affects, all of which affect the various ingredients of the treatment relationship—namely, transference, therapeutic alliance, and countertransference. Aspects of nonverbal communication, such as body language, eye contacts and eye signals, facial expressions, touching, and the like, also have different meanings in different cultures. Some cultures, defined as "high-context" cultures, will rely more heavily on the nonverbal context than on the verbal context.

Chin (1994) recommends that greater attention be paid to nonverbal contextual communication. Simplistic, immediate acceptance of silence as compliance will only produce flawed interpersonal exchanges between client and clinician. "For an Asian client, silence cannot be interpreted as agreement if the client is not contradicting the therapist to be polite. For a Black client, silence may represent suspiciousness and threat of challenging an authority figure" (p. 211).

Of crucial importance in culturally competent and responsive therapy is the need to verbalize the issues of race and ethnicity in the therapeutic relationship and in the transference. In particular, Chin (1994) has stressed the need to support clients' positive identifications with aspects of their racial and ethnic identity, to correct for the devalued aspects of race and ethnicity in U.S. society.

COUNTERTRANSFERENCE

General Overview and Definitions

"Countertransference," like "transference," is an overused term. Commonly, it covers any and all feelings and reactions of the therapist in response to the patient. Some believe that countertransference arises not out of a client's behavior alone, but from unconscious and preconscious forces within the therapist that cause the therapist to react to the patient in ways that are inappropriate to the current reality of the therapeutic relationships. Such unrealistic, unprovoked realities are viewed as displacements from the therapist's significant early relationships with his or her own siblings and parents. Giovacchini (1985) differs and offers a far broader definition:

> I believe countertransference is ubiquitous; it is found in every analytic interaction in the same way that transference is. Everything a therapist or a patient thinks, feels, or does can be viewed [as] being on a hierarchical spectrum, one end dominated by unconscious, primary process elements, and the other end dominated by reality-oriented secondary process factors. When a patient directs his feelings toward the therapist, the primary process elements of the spectrum represents transference, and in a similar fashion that part of the analyst's responses that stems primarily from the more primitive levels of his psyche can be viewed as countertransference. (p. 45)

Some clinicians make distinctions along Giovacchini's spectrum, designating reality-oriented factors as "counterreactions" and those that emanate out of unconscious variables as "countertransference." Most clinicians recognize that when a counterreaction is used defensively, it can interrupt or disrupt the clinician's analyzing function, because it "activates a developmental residue and creates or revives unconscious conflict, anxiety and defensiveness" (Marcus, 1980, p. 286). When it is not used defensively, it can be a valuable diagnostic tool and effective treatment response, in which a therapist is led to reflect and undertake a frank examination of his or her aroused feelings to avoid or resolve various therapeutic impasses or stalemates. There are appropriate and all-but-universal counterreactions to specific clients: those who are very impulsive, acting out, highly narcissistic, extremely aggressive, unmotivated and resistive, or suicidal. Such clients arouse understandable anxiety, fears, and frustrations in all therapists (Mishne, 1997).

There is also naturally a wide variation in a clinician's fit with different clients. One cannot work equally effectively with all of one's clients. "Rather than viewing treatability only in terms of the patient's limitations, it is more realistic to consider the patient/therapist relationship as the axis that determines treatability. A patient may not be treatable by a particular therapist, but that does not make that patient untreatable" (Giovacchini, 1985, p. 450).

Some patients provoke anger, rejection, and hostile demands for compliance; others cause therapists to feel anxious, overwhelmed, helpless, or ashamed. A patient who is productive and promising may please and gratify a therapist, who unconsciously misuses that patient as a narcissistic extension. Signs of countertransference problems are the therapist's lateness, boredom, overinvolvement, noncontained fear and/or anger, mistakes about scheduling, and the like. The clinician must be self-observing and self-aware, and seek appropriate sources of help and support in order to minimize the potentially problematic impact such reactions may otherwise have. Supervision, consultation, and personal treatment help the therapist to stay in touch with and control his or her unconscious and preconscious early conflicts and prejudices, and properly modulate conscious behaviors and response. "The goal is to provide a safe holding environment, one that is characterized by restraint, appropriate containment of drive expression, attunement, an absence of nihilistic pessimism and a conscious sense of concern and compassion, based on the clinician's ability to [draw on the client's] history" (Mishne, 1997, p. 115). This enables the clinician to see and be sensitive to the patient's earlier injuries and pain, which have produced unpleasant primitive defenses such as denial, projection, splitting, and externalization.

More Recent Perspectives on Countertransference

Hanna (1998) reviews more recent perspectives on countertransference, and states that under "the influence of the Kleinian and British Independent Schools of object relations and the Cultural School in the United States, an expanded view of countertransference developed: the [early] totalistic position, [which] emphasized the use of the therapist's total emotional reaction to the patient for diagnostic and treatment purposes" (p. 4). This perspective maintained a positivist view of countertransference, which requires containment so as not to contaminate the patient's transference distortion. A more recent totalistic perspective, foreshadowed by Bion's (1955) view of the patient's projective idealizations and the clinician's containment functions, is a decisive new step in viewing therapy as a two-person interpersonal process. Sandler (1976, p. 4) emphasized the need for clinicians to be aware of their behavioral responsiveness, and of the potential danger in complying with the roles they are cast into by patients.

According to Hanna (1998), the intersubjective perspective on countertransference, which is closely associated with self psychology, shifts the focus from the therapist's intrapsychic dynamics to the here-and-now interplay between the differently organized subjective worlds of the observer and the observed, with introspection and empathy as central to the method of observation (Atwood & Stolorow, 1984). British analysts Winnicott, Heimann, Bion, Rocker, and Rosenfeld, especially Bion, are credited with reframing projective identification toward a greater emphasis on the interpersonal. However, Hanna also notes that within all schools of psychoanalytic theory, analytically oriented clinicians have recently begun placing greater emphasis on the here-and-now and on an interpersonal view of therapy. The clinician is no longer viewed as a blank screen or detached observer, but rather as a participant/observer. "Greater acceptance of the irreducible subjectivity of the therapist has led to an overall democratization of the therapeutic dyad" (Hanna, 1998, p. 12). Accordingly, many classically trained analysts have surrendered time-honored practice rules and have moved away from the traditional emphasis on the therapist's anonymity. Rinik (1995) believes that we clinicians need to move beyond our traditional ideas about self-disclosure, and openly share and communicate any and everything that in our view might be helpful to our patients. Earlier, Gill (1982) recommended that a clinician interpret the transference as something that is not displacement, but rather refers to something that has actually occurred between the patient and clinician. This can include a therapist's counterreactions, and/or mistakes or failures (e.g., a therapeutic rupture).

Others recommend determining and sharing the meaning of countertransference reactions and the impact of these on patients (Bacal, 1985; Balint, 1968; Newman, 1985). Also emphasizing self-disclosure are those who follow a contemporary social-constructivist perspective. Speaking for this model, Hoffman (1996) notes that he has "shared quite a bit with the patient, regarding my background and my own attitudes and conflicts; sometimes, having those things on the table gives the patient the chance to see the relativity of the analyst's point of view to the analyst's own experience and history" (p. 132).

Clearly, self-disclosure and the provision of spontaneous feedback both characterize the contemporary, more interpersonally oriented therapist, and are newer ways of managing the countertransference. Older techniques, especially the emphasis on neutrality and abstinence from action, are increasingly criticized and viewed as interfering with the therapist's authenticity. Some clinicians dedicated to newer two-person intersubjective perspectives seem "bent on sniffing out and totally eradicating any personal tendency to be the arbiter of reality and [instead focus] on appearing totally authentic and transparent to their patients" (Hanna, 1998, p. 19). A more conservative perspective cautions that self-disclosure should not be an imperative; rather, it should be offered judiciously, on a case-by-case basis, since some patients cannot use language symbolically. Other patients may find their therapists' self-revelations exploitive, seductive, and/or critical and judgmental (Hanna, 1998; Mitchell, 1997). Some clients may experience such sharing as due to a therapist's narcissistic need to be at center stage, or may interpret it as meaning that they, the patients, are no longer of interest to their therapists, who have lost the ability to listen and follow their material (i.e., the patients' affects, moods, feelings, and needs).

I concur with the reservations raised by Hanna (1998) about universal self-disclosure by therapists: "Therapist self-revelation is not necessarily reflective of a true capacity for authenticity, relatedness and intimacy. Surely, an a priori imperative that a therapist should self-reveal is incompatible with authenticity. There is often a strained quality in therapists who technically employ self-revelation in psychotherapy" (p. 19). Self-disclosure must not be viewed all on its own as a necessary technique, intervention, or parameter, but rather in the context of the specific treatment relationship. How long have the patient and clinician worked together? What is the history of their relationship? What is its emotional tone? How good is the dyadic fit?

Despite the variety of stylistic approaches and techniques recommended by various contemporary interpersonal therapists, intersubjectivity theory expands our understanding of the interplay between transference and countertransference. Moving away from the adhesion to objective reality, it has shown clinicians the importance of subjective reality and the need for clinical investigation from a perspective within a subjective world. The optimal therapeutic stance is an attitude of sustained empathic inquiry, which "contributes to the formation of an intersubjective situation in which the patient increasingly comes to believe that his most profound emotional states and needs can be understood in depth" (Stolorow, Brandchaft, & Atwood, 1987, p. 10).

Shane and Shane (1998) review the efforts of a number of significant thinkers/researchers to define the therapist's optimal stance in the clinical situation. They introduce their own concept of "optimal restraint," and they note that Bacal advocates "optimal responsiveness"; Stolorow and colleagues, "attunement to affect states"; Basch, "attention to pathological affect states"; and Beebe and Lachmann, "attention to patterns of mutual and self-regulation." These offerings of the followers and extenders of self psychology do not minimize Kohut's emphasis on "empathy," however. Kohut considered empathy "a value neutral method of observation attuned to the inner life of man" (1984, p. 395). Clearly, empathy is a critical ingredient in countertransference, and accurate empathy is composed of both affective and cognitive components. Empathy is not used to satisfy or gratify the patient's needs, nor is it the same as sympathy or support. "Rather, empathy informs the individual as to what is needed or yearned for by the other" (Lynch, 1991, p. 16). Kohut (1978) summarized his understanding of empathy with the following propositions:

> 1) Empathy, the recognition of the self in the other, is an indispensable tool of observation without which vast areas of human life, including man's behavior in the social field remain unintelligible. 2) Empathy, the expansion of the self to include the other, constitutes a powerful psychological bond between individuals, which, perhaps more than love, the expression and sublimation of the sexual drive, counteracts man's destructiveness against his fellows. 3) Empathy, the accepting, confirming and understanding human echo evoked by the self, is a psychological nutriment without which human life as we know it and cherish it could not be sustained. (p. 84)

In the context of the treatment relationship within a self-psychological perspective, the therapist must strive for empathic immersion, in order to gain a real understanding of each client's demands, hopes, fears, ambitions, and symptomatic behavior. "The theory of self psychology removes the focus from the patient's faulty functioning in favor of learning to understand the underlying structure responsible for the faulty functioning" (Basch, 1980, p. 409).

Following the achievement of understanding, interpretations are offered to assist in structure building—that is, providing a compensatory structure for a client whose development was interrupted or thwarted by traumatic empathic failure in early life (Basch, 1980). Although better cognition and insight may occur, a major goal of treatment is to open a path of empathy between self and selfobject, and to deepen the client's capacity for self-acceptance. A further treatment goal is the development of a cohesive self, through the process Kohut called "transmuting internalization." Transmuting internalization occurs as clients "develop a capacity to accept the hurts that are caused by failures of optimal responses by important others" (Solomon, 1991, p. 132). Kohut (1984, p. 78) viewed treatment as a "correctional emotional experience," and it is generally agreed that the expanded theoretical constructs of self psychology have been particularly useful in countertransference-based work with more fragile populations.

Countertransference Issues with Clients of Color

As the preceding discussion indicates, in recent years there has been an "increasing openness of the investigative spirit in its revisions and expansion of [clinical] theory and less self-conscious defensiveness about orthodoxy of tradition. Innovation in technical interventions can now be discussed in a freer atmosphere" (Lazar, 1998, p. 214). Nowhere is such innovation needed more than in the mental health field's efforts to provide effective service to an ever-growing population of culturally diverse patients. Because of the demographic changes described in Chapters 1 and 2, "the ascendancy of cultural pluralism needs to be reflected in the delivery of mental health services" (Comas-Díaz & Greene, 1994a, p. 3). And therapists' use of the countertransference in their work with clients is no exception to this rule.

　　Chin (1994) summarizes findings regarding matched racial minority dyads, that is, therapists of color often become overidentified with their clients of color, and thus may be oversensitive to racial overtones in their interpretation of dynamic content. As a result, they may overprotect their clients against such overtones by avoiding appropriate confrontation of intrapsychic dynamics. Clinicians of color may also overemphasize policy and social change strategies to deal with racism, thus neglecting the interventions of introspection needed by their clients. Along with potential overidentification with clients of color is an often-noted mistaken underdiagnosis of psychopathology. However, Chin also notes a different type of problem—namely, that minority therapists' adherence to majority values may cause them to disregard aspects of their own and their clients' culture:

> Therapists of color can also internalize biases and distortions related to race, culture, and gender prevalent in our society. Since most are trained in Western models of psychotherapy, they can support culturally dystonic values and strategies as therapeutic goals. For example, they may support women of color in assertively confronting their husbands; while they may view this [as] acculturation, liberation, and so on, such confrontations could serve to emasculate these men according to cultural norms. On the other hand, women of color may over-identify with cultural norms and support culturally prescribed gender roles, to the detriment of self-esteem and actualization. (p. 212)

Despite the various pitfalls for some matched racial minority dyads, in other situations the match can be a boom in regard to transference and countertransference issues. Some clinicians of color can use this variable in their self-identity to identify appropriately with clients of color, and thereby to facilitate a strong alliance. The clients' gains are noteworthy in these circumstances; they often include better self-esteem, improved ego functioning, better social and familial relationships, enhanced job performance, and better modulation of drive expression (i.e., aggression and sexual impulses).

White therapists working with clients of color may be unaware of cultural nuances, or may lack an empathic comprehension of what such clients have endured, helplessly and ragefully, in frightening racial encounters. Often countertransference phenomena, like transference phenomena (as discussed earlier in this chapter), will be associated with the dynamics of power differences between client and therapist. Racial and/or ethnic differences between client and therapist often cause anxiety; thus it is not uncommon for white therapists to minimize the cultural, racial, and (if present) gender differences between themselves and their clients of color. When white therapists claim or assume that wants, needs, and problems are universal, they often lose sight of or inappropriately minimize differences, or "rely on racial and cultural stereotypes that result in a superficial interpretation of cultural phenomena" (Chin, 1994, p. 212). Some white clinicians can overdiagnose psychopathology. In other cases, unmodulated emotional reactions to clients' lives, or invasive inquisitiveness about clients' families or cultural norms, cause clients of color to feel misunderstood and not at all valued or trusted. White therapists' conscious or unconscious racism can result in interpretations and diagnoses that demean their minority clients and convey only stereotypic expectations of the clients' behavior; if clients indeed respond to these expectations by behaving stereotypically (in a sort of self-fulfilling prophecy), this may be countered by inappropriate displays of power on the clinician's part.

However, empathic and attuned white therapists can be most effective and facilitative in working with clients of color. Such a therapist's ease in acknowledging cultural differences, as well as admitting ignorance about a client's culture and a wish to correct this ignorance, can promote a client's feeling of safety in sharing his or her personal history and cultural identity. As the therapeutic work in such a dyad progresses, culturally sensitive countertransference requires a reframing of therapeutic issues within the client's world view, rather than an evaluation of the client's customs in contrast with the therapist's majority culture. In particular, reframing therapeutic outcomes to be syntonic with the client's cultural values will be important. This may require taking new perspectives about family rules and roles, as well as age-appropriate tasks and achievements.

Splitting, which is traditionally viewed as a developmentally primitive defense, may be a useful defense for bicultural individuals who live in environments where the values and practices of both cultures can be discrepant and contradictory. "It is not uncommon for bicultural individuals to maintain separate and distinct selves syntonic with different cultures" (Chin, 1994, pp. 213–214). In considering the processes of immigration and acculturation, Chin (1988) underscores the stressors that takes their toll on mental health and status, particularly in women of color. Other authors note the strength and flexibility entailed in achieving and maintaining a bicultural identity. Comas-Díaz and Minrath (1985), for example, reflect on the strengths needed to overcome difficulties en route to the attainment of optimal and positive self-identity.

Root (1985) notes the limitations of present models for optimal ethnic identity among biracial individuals. Commonly, biracial individuals struggle with ambiguous and marginal socioethnic status. Biracial clients, especially women, often present in psychotherapy with feelings of estrangement, loss, and alienation. In such cases, acculturation no longer is the sole goal pursued; rather, clinicians and clients seek to reinforce the strength of a bicultural identity.

As this discussion has emphasized, culturally competent management of cultural countertransference requires communicating across cultures. Wu (1987) stresses the need for a cultural empathy that empowers the patient as a partner in the therapeutic process. He emphasizes understanding the patient within his or her cultural context. Reframing psychotherapy from this anthropological perspective facilitates viewing cultural phenomena in psychotherapy as different, rather than deviant.

Ethnocultural transference and countertransference phenomena are best handled within a system, institution, or agency that is culturally competent (Perez Foster, 1998a). Cross, Bazron, Dennis, and Isaacs (1989) note five essential elements to assist a clinician or an agency in becoming more culturally competent: (1) valuing diversity; (2) having the capacity for cultural self-assessment; (3) being conscious of the dynamics inherent in the interaction of cultures; (4) having institutional cultural knowledge; and (5) developing adaptation to diversity.

CASE OF CARLA: EXAMPLE OF TRANSFERENCE AND COUNTERTRANSFERENCE IN THE TREATMENT OF AN AMERICAN-BORN HISPANIC WOMAN

Development, Family, and Psychosocial History

Carla and I have worked together most productively for an extraordinary length of time. We have known each other for more than a decade, and have shared two extensive courses of treatment. (The break in treatment was necessitated by Carla's having to be out of town following her receipt of a prestigious award for a year of advanced training, after completion of her graduate studies.)

Carla was referred to me by a therapist in the Midwest she had worked with during her adolescence. She had initiated her first treatment contact while in high school, due to her feelings of low self-esteem and severe insecurity. Her mother was also in counseling, and supported and assisted Carla in her pursuit of therapy. Later, Carla resumed contact with her first therapist, since she experienced panic attacks in college and could not return to school after her freshman year. After being on leave from college for 7 months, she returned to school and began to work with a psychiatrist in her college community, who provided medication and nondirective psychotherapy over a 4-year period. Two years after graduation from college, Carla joined the Peace Corps; however, she again suffered such intense panic attacks that she had to leave the Peace Corps and return home, finding herself fragmenting and completely overwhelmed. After 9 months at home and in therapy again, she moved east, found work, and sought reentry into treatment, fearing the reappearance of anxiety and panic attacks. She also was seeking relief from and help with long-standing bulimia nervosa, a disorder that first appeared in college.

Joining friends from college, Carla was able to find affordable housing and an interesting job at a realtor's office. She was assigned to work on a development project for a specialty shopping center devoted to the arts, antiques, and the like. She assessed this as having more potential for advancement than her prior secretarial job at a brokerage house. She had felt humiliated, invisible, and rudely treated when working as a secretary.

Carla reported that she endlessly worried and always felt anxious or depressed, with extreme mood swings that she attempted to control or soothe via food; the result had become a painful pattern of overeating, vomiting, and inordinate weight gain. At the time we began treatment, Carla was grossly overweight, weighing close to 180 pounds. Carla said that she had never been at ease with boyfriends. Her weight gains commonly occurred as a response to too much attention from males, and/or following the conclusion of a relationship. Her mother, in her view, was pressing her to get married and thus not to repeat the mother's history of marrying late (at age 32, after leaving her family in Mexico in shame over her single status). Carla's mother had a bookkeeping degree from a junior college, and she had worked since Carla and her siblings began attending school full time. Carla was the oldest of three, having a sister 2 years younger and a brother 5 years younger. Her sister, a college graduate and married, was a secretary, and her brother had graduated from a good engineering school.

For years Carla had felt closer to her mother and sister than to her dad and brother. She had only perfunctory phone contact with the men of the family, whereas she was excessively overinvolved with and made very frequent phone calls to her sister and mother. Carla worried about trying to meet appropriate young men she could date; she commonly first got overexcited about, and then overanxious about and/or overly depreciating of, any potential boyfriend. She deplored not attracting more personable and appealing young men, even when she was slim and attractive, and acknowledged her own self-consciousness and anxiety as deterrents. She viewed her mother as becoming more and more traditionally "Latin" in pressing her daughters to marry. Carla rarely had contact with Latino males. She was very denigrating about their reputed *machismo*, promiscuity, and tendency to be less than reliable and responsible for their families. Her own father did not conform to her stereotyped portrait; rather, he was responsible and loyal, but also taciturn, unaffectionate, highly critical, and hot-tempered. He was described as endlessly complaining that his children were not appreciative of what he provided them, and that his daughters were too casual about their studies. His complaints about Carla's mother were said to be mean, small-minded, and endless. The parents were not affectionate and used to argue a lot. More recently, they seem to have become closer and somewhat less argumentative. Carla told me, "My dad's still an immigrant, constantly using the hard times of his youth as his point of reference." Her dad had been born in Ecuador, the 7th of 13 children. Despite the paternal grandfather's education, family size reduced them to a near-poverty level; this nevertheless did not inhibit Carla's dad and his siblings from seeking and obtaining college-level education, and entering such professions as engineering.

Carla's parents had upper-middle-class earning capacity, and accordingly sought such a neighborhood in which to raise their family. With three other Hispanic couples, they purchased homes in one of the more affluent suburbs of their large Midwestern city. Because the other families had so few children (only one had a daughter close in age to Carla and her sister), Carla and her siblings were a real minority in their school. Carla said that although she appreciated attending excellent schools and having a nice home and yard in an attractive suburb, she would have preferred anything to what was provided in her parents' search for an optimal socioeconomic and academic environment for their children. Things were fairly comfortable until adolescence, when Carla and her siblings were no longer routinely included in any social events or parties with their peers. Earlier, there had seemed to be acceptance, warmth, and inclusion of the children in the predominantly Jewish community. However, Carla's parents remained unintegrated. When issues of dating and the like arose during Carla's and her siblings' adolescence, the invitations seemed to cease.

At the onset of therapy and for many years, Carla demonstrated self-depreciation and group depreciation in regard to her Latina/ Hispanic American identity (Atkinson et al., 1998; Ruiz, 1990). Carla felt that she and her siblings had all suffered from being so alone in their affluent suburb, and wished that her parents had lived beneath their socioeconomic status, had settled in a more Latino community, or had migrated back to their countries of origin (where

Carla believed she would have felt more secure with a kinship support system).

In college, she was flooded by overtures and attention from well-to-do Hispanic youths sent to the States for academic and professional gains beyond those available in their various South American countries. When Carla's weight was appropriate, she was (and is) a strikingly lovely young woman, with beautiful features, a fair complexion, and dark hair. She was operated on in high school for scoliosis, and there was no sign of the curvature of the spine, which was all but perfectly corrected. Because of her natural beauty, she did attract a great deal of attention—"too much attention to handle"—in college, and thereupon she hid behind a curtain of shyness and weight increase of more than 60 and 70 pounds. She'd had no dating or socializing experience in high school, due to her recuperation from back surgery and her problems with social acceptance in her high school. She did not retain any connection with peers until she graduated from college, worked, and made more meaningful and enduring friendships (which still continue). Carla's shyness was often her predominant affect in new situations (e.g., upon beginning a new job). Carla had no close friends who shared her Hispanic background. She also had no special closeness with Hispanic colleagues at her place of work.

Over the years, Carla and I have worked very well on a biweekly basis. Treatment is provided at a scaled-down fee, given her low earnings for so long, her part-time graduate school attendance, and her still-existent college and graduate school loans. When we began to work together, she demonstrated poor money management, much like her poor management of food. She'd overbuy and overspend on impractical items (e.g., clothing and cosmetics) that were excessively expensive for a young person working as a low-level secretary and/or a realtor's assistant. Once Carla got a grip on her spending habits, she veered to the other extreme, becoming not only careful but penurious. In recent years, she has finally found a sensible and realistic balance in the management of her monies—bills, student loans, and the like. She now takes pride in her self-sufficiency and self-support.

Her management of foods has been a more problematic issue. Typically, she would maintain rigid control over eating until she encountered some stressor; this would be followed by bingeing, regression, and relapse. In the last 2½ years, she has made great progress in managing food and sustaining a normal, healthy weight. A major focus in therapy was paternal intrusiveness about food at the family dinner hour. Bullied to eat meat, Carla developed an aversion to it and hid her meat portions in a decorative centerpiece at the table, which then had to be cleaned and emptied for the next subterfuge. This routine went on for years, and only in the last couple of years has Carla been able to purchase, prepare, and consume meat, fish, and poultry. She never considered herself a vegetarian, but in fact she did confine herself to carbohydrates and some canned vegetables. She has learned in recent years to eat and enjoy more balanced meals, rather than replicating her depressed mother, who struggled with food preparation for her family in the face of her nonexistent culinary skills.

Carla no longer mirrors her mother, with whom she originally claimed she felt as one, fearful at the mere idea of separation and individuation. She's been able to move out of the primary relationship that so tightly bound her and her mother, to make an authentic connection with her father. Feeling relaxed with both parents has enhanced her self-esteem. Having more rapport with her dad does not feel disloyal to her mother today, as it did in the past. In fact, Carla recently took a trip to Ecuador with her dad and reveled in connecting with his relatives more closely than before.

Cultural Identity Issues for Carla and Her Family

Lu and colleagues (1995) note that the best way to learn about patients' ethnicity (especially when it differs from that of clinicians) is to ask the patients to describe their grandparents' and parents' country (of countries) of origin, religion, primary language, and traditional roles and skills. Over time, I was able to learn many details from Carla about her father's and mother's histories, religious observances, roles and values, migrations, and the like.

Cultural identity includes not just the fact that one is a member of a particular group; it also includes the dimension of "cultural identity development," which refers to how a culturally diverse individual sees him- or herself in respect to the host culture (Ivey, Ivey, & Simek-Morgan, 1993). Carla's parents did not emphasize their cultural background while Carla was growing up. For example, they did not frequently or routinely visit their families of origin, despite maintaining ongoing contact with their relatives. Carla believes that this was a mistaken economy, and that it served to dilute Carla's and her siblings' ethnic identity (which she has only relatively recently reasserted). Although Spanish was spoken in her family of origin, it was somewhat depreciated by her father, who deplored her mother's poor command of English. Carla's parents shared Hispanic origins, but came from different countries and had different levels of acculturation to life in the United States. Her Ecuadorean father was professionally more acculturated, functioning as a competent engineer in a sizable firm, in contrast to his Mexican wife, a homemaker who gradually sought part-time employment as a bookkeeper in a neighborhood-based nursing home—a place where she enjoyed working, despite her lack of integration with (and only marginal ties with) other employees.

Despite Carla's mother's shyness and numerous anxieties and overreactions, Carla has described her as quietly and gradually becoming increasingly self-assertive. Carla attributes this to the mother's own long course of supportive psychotherapy, her employment, and her independent management of a considerable portion of her earnings. Carla views her mother as becoming, in a complex fashion, less submissive and more acculturated (to American women's rights, etc.) in the home than her dad. Her father formerly attempted to maintain a *machismo*, more dominant position; this has only lessened in recent years under the impact of grandparenthood, his own retirement, and his recent joining with his wife to offer support via some child care for Carla's sister's child. Carla views her own improved relationship with her dad as another explanation for her father's improved familial stance with his wife and three now-adult children.

Although women in general and Hispanic women in particular are noted as having more positive attitudes toward counseling, and are more likely to disclose their thoughts and feelings to a counselor (Zimmerman & Sodowsky, 1993), Carla's father has recently sought some supportive therapy (in response to her and her mother's urging) for help with his low-level depression since his recent retirement. Indeed, in Carla's family of origin, all but her brother have sought and benefited from therapy.

Carla often observes that her siblings have no discernible validation or sense of affirmation of their ethnic heritage. This is noted in contrast to her own ever-increasing positive feelings about her Hispanic heritage, which she reflects as an outcome of our work together. She has recently married and has chosen to retain her Hispanic maiden name; she has also dedicated herself to working with Hispanic clients, using Spanish. She often reflects ruefully on her prior sense of self-consciousness and shame about her Latina heritage. I have consciously and realistically felt and demonstrated real interest in Carla's history, and in her family of origin's immigration and acculturation experience. Ours has been a relationship of genuine warmth, trust, and rapport, and Carla states that my interest in and respect for her culture gave her permission to look at, learn about, and identify positively with her heritage.

DISCUSSION OF ETHNIC/CULTURAL ISSUES IN THE TRANSFERENCE AND COUNTERTRANSFERENCE PHENOMENA WITH CARLA

Comas-Díaz and Jacobsen (1991) enumerate a range of possible interethnic transference responses, from overfriendliness or denial of ethnic and cultural differences on the one hand to mistrust, suspicion, hostility, or ambivalence on the other. In addition, interethnic transference often results in a patient's being overly compliant and overly pleasing in an attempt to negate or negotiate a perceived power differential.

Carla often referred to her adolescent and early adult years as "the time I wanted to be Jewish," in order to fit into the peer culture of her family's place of residence. All her life, she has had Jewish peers and a high percentage of Jewish therapists and teachers, and as a teenager and young woman she emphasized what she saw as positive Jewish ethnic and cultural values. These included close-knit families; egalitarian marriages; equal opportunities and rights for sons and daughters; high priority on educational and professional achievements, civic responsibility, and philanthropy; artistic and aesthetic sophistication; high-income achievements; and so forth. In our early work together, she dated a Jewish young man, and avidly fantasized about their eventually marrying and her eagerly converting to Judaism. Prior to our work together, I had no experience with clients so openly envious of my Jewish identity and ethnic background, and so overly respectful in demeanor. Initially I had to struggle to handle my own early interethnic countertransference, best characterized as a low-level degree of discomfort, guilt, and pity in response to Carla's self-denigration and overidealization of a Jewish identity. These feelings were intensified because of my own sense of security, power, and pleasure in my Jewish identity (which I describe in greater detail in Chapter 6).

I was concerned about Carla's compliant stance with me, as well as in most relationships in her life. I recognized her problems with handling her anger, and her habitual patterns of oversubmission and overaccommodation to others; these seemed to have some traditional cultural components, but went even beyond what most Hispanic cultures prescribe for women. In the context of the transference and the lengthy treatment process, as the relationship deepened, Carla developed trust and worked very hard, and was successful in making significant and substantial changes. I utilized techniques of understanding, explanation, and interpretation; these flowed from my efforts to immerse myself empathically in Carla's context (particularly her cultural context), to give me a depth of emotional understanding of her hopes, demands, ambitions, struggles, and symptomatic behaviors. "To put it another way, the theory of self psychology removes the focus from the patient's faulty functioning in favor of learning to understand the underlying structure responsible for the faulty functioning" (Basch, 1980, p. 409). This differs greatly from the common classic position of critical confrontation of the patient's evasions, demands, and actions, which often threatens the treatment process. As noted earlier in this chapter, the goal is to provide structure building as a consequence of optimal responsiveness. "Structure" in this sense refers not to the classic psychic structure of ego, superego, and id, but rather to a deficit-filling or cohesion-confirming structure of the self, which compensates for the earlier interruption or thwarting of development (Basch, 1980).

I was able to convey to Carla my emotional sense of her pains and hurts from early childhood on, when she felt shy and embarrassed in peer groups by her mother's lack of facility in speaking English, and was wounded by her mother's lack of inclusion by other mothers in the neighborhood in the arrangement of children's play dates. I felt a palpable awareness of young Carla's shy and tongue-tied stance on the fringe of this or that peer group, or her frozen, hurt response once she realized she'd not been invited to this or that Bar Mitzvah party. Similarly, she could convey her past discomfort about her scoliosis and curtailment of swimming and water ballet activities in high school. Equally vivid were her accounts of her panic attacks (which had caused her to leave college and the Peace Corps), and her shame about her overeating binges followed by vomiting purges.

We both believe that the exceptional rapport between us enabled Carla to become more verbally expressive and self-aware. What follows is an excerpt from the journal she began to keep in regard to her struggles with bulimia, whereby, over time, she could talk out rather than act out the impulse to binge and gorge herself on vast quantities of inappropriate food.

What is so difficult about not eating to stifle a feeling is that you have to feel the feeling. It seems that every day there are five or six different episodes of feelings that are accustomed to being dealt with by a blondie [a type of brownie] or granola bars. When that food is not available it feels like I'm going to pop or break. I'm not used to feeling these feelings.

Without the food I feel I am without armor; I have no defense against my life. I cannot have a "time out" evening or week(!) I have to experience the frustration or anxiety, try to find the root of it, and then try to either remedy the circumstance causing the feeling or simply let the feeling pass without doing anything else.

I have no practice at feeling loneliness, anger, frustration. I am sure I knew how to handle these feelings at one point, but it seems like years that I have felt lonely, months since I've been angry and recognized it. Frustration? I don't think I've ever let frustration come and go without running to or thinking about escaping with food.

This is what I am all about. This is how my adulthood has passed—a battle of stifling feelings and emotions. Maybe out of fear of not knowing how to handle the feelings, maybe out of fear of pain, that they will hurt too much.

I don't know. All I know is that I cannot continue running away from life, although every day there is a minute or hour or hours when I ache to and mull over going home, bag of ice cream, scone and whatnot in hand, and settling down on the sofa with the television on all evening. This is how I have numbed myself and consequently I have not developed the ability to tolerate feelings and to tolerate the inconsistencies of life.

I am behind in this school of adult living. What grade am I in? How long will it take me to catch up or to at least get to a higher grade? Am I going to have a headache every day? Are we talking months or years?

Wednesday	Tuesday
final exam	spending money
not going out during lunch time	rudeness at Macy's

HIV   being a perfect secretary
Thanksgiving

*As I write down these stressors, I think to myself, "I want to
erase everything so that I don't pop, so that I don't suddenly
jump up and run down to the corner grocery store and buy a
box of crackers." Sometimes I feel that the feelings will continue to accumulate until they reach a breaking point and that I
have no control over the explosion that will result from reaching that breaking point. I have no control, no say, no voice, no
power. Something else determines my life when I know as a
sane adult that I can control a great deal more of my life than I
have been doing.*

As Carla has realized that she can control more of her life than
she was formerly doing, over time she has made impressive gains
and changes. She no longer suffers from bulimia or panic attacks.
She has been able to find a most gratifying profession, and to put
herself through a rigorous, demanding, and expensive graduate
school master's degree program in social work. Following receipt of
her master's degree, she received a prestigious fellowship for a year's
advanced study. She has taken great pleasure in finally achieving all
age-appropriate developmental milestones. Namely, she has developed a personal identity that includes a strong sense of her Latina
cultural heritage; she has established a professional identity; and,
finally (which proved most elusive), she has found a satisfying romantic partner, married, and had a child. She is amazed and thrilled
at being a successful mother to a contented and responsive infant
son. Equally thrilling is the ease with which she has managed food
and weight issues, even while pregnant and since the birth of her
child. In keeping with her and her husband's secure financial situation, she will return to work only on a part-time basis. Being offered
a prestigious new position in her new neighborhood has further enhanced Carla's ever-growing sense of self-esteem, which she believes
is the outcome of her hard work and her very successful experience
in treatment.

When examined through a self-psychological lens, Carla's final transference configuration appears to have moved beyond ethnic/cultural transference phenomena, and rather is best described as an idealizing transference. As noted earlier in this chapter, the idealizing transference (Kohut, 1977) develops from insufficiently responded-to early needs for merger with a strong, calm parental figure. In treatment, the therapist is experienced as omniscient, omnipotent, and perfect. Kohut (1977) cautioned therapists not to rebuff or reject patients' idealizations, in contrast to classic theory, but instead to show greater tolerance of idealizations and deidealizations. Likewise, idealizations can appear in clinicians' counterreactions and countertransferences. It is essential that a countertransferential idealization not be a rigid stance, demanding continued perfection and/or idealizations from the patient; rather, it should be one that can reflect back great respect, compassion, regard, and even "love," which Freud stated was the essence of cure.

It is not hard for me to admire, respect, and love Carla, and to find joy in sharing in her accomplishments. Her very words, in one of the many notes sent over the years, demonstrate her idealization and regard—which I believe I return with great love and respect, via an idealizing countertransference.

Dear Dr. Mishne,

In the ten years that we have known each other, you have been my guide, my friend, my confidant, and my ideal object. Your professionalism and nurturing manner will not be equaled by anyone who passes through my life. Of this I am certain. You know me and have been instrumental in my development. My self-awareness and strengths are tributes to you and to your steady presence and support. I admire you, care for you, am in awe of you and hold you in a special place in my heart and in my self.

Carla

Carla's note appears to be in essential agreement with self psychologist Marian Tolpin's (1983) view of the treatment process as a reciprocal exchange between patient and analyst, which she calls a "corrective development dialogue" involving "the establishment, interpretation and working through of a new transference edition of the self–selfobject unit [between child and parent]" (p. 366).

THE REAL RELATIONSHIP

In an extraordinary little book titled *Freud and Man's Soul*, Bruno Bettelheim (1983) attempted to correct what he viewed as the mistranslation of Freud and many of his most important psychoanalytic concepts. Bettelheim's thesis was that the English translations of Freud are seriously flawed, and that as a result, erroneous conclusions have been reached both about Freud the man and also about the process of psychoanalysis. Bettelheim's goal was to show the humane Freud, whom he presented as a "humanist in the best sense of the word. His greatest concern was with man's inner most being, to which he most frequently referred through the use of a metaphor—man's soul—because the word 'soul' evokes so many emotional connotations" (p. xi). Quoting from one of Freud's letters to Jung, Bettelheim stated, "Psychoanalysis is in essence a cure through love" (p. xi).

Seemingly the abounding mistranslations and misunderstanding of Freud have led traditional analytically oriented clinicians to adopt a rigid posture of a blank screen, unaffected by a patient's verbal and behavioral manifestations. Adherents to this mode are silent, impassive, and unresponsive to all they hear or see.

> The result is that too often perfectly decent, friendly, curious and helpful people act like robots when they begin to function as psychotherapists. They literally wonder whether they should smile or shake hands upon greeting a patient the first time, worry whether such behavior might already "contaminate" the field, as if a relationship between two living beings could be reduced to the artificial atmosphere of a physics or chemistry laboratory. (Basch, 1980, p. 4)

This misunderstanding of Freud's teachings has created what Basch (1980) called the "dogma and myth" of the therapist's anonymity—a stance that is particularly contraindicated in cross-cultural psychotherapy. Basch recommended injection of a personal note whenever appropriate in all treatment relationships. Many patients, particularly those in treatment with a clinician of a different race or ethnic group, generally cannot tolerate a passive, silent, or stilted approach; it creates a sense of discomfort, distrust, and expectations of criticism. This is commonly the reason for such patients' intense anxiety, increased defensiveness, distrust, or even premature flight from therapy.

Alexander (1963) was one of the first to challenge the neutrality of the analyst. He stated emphatically that the analyst's values are subtly learned by the patient through verbal and nonverbal communications, and that the experience of genuineness, warmth, and respect is a corrective emotional experience with a real person. Marmor (1982) emphasized the value of empathic warmth, attentive listening, and active participation in the treatment process. These modifications of "classic neutral technique" are essential in cross-cultural treatment.

The interpersonal interactional role is suggested by Blanck and Blanck (1979a) in their description of a therapist as "development reorganizer of the patient's subphase inadequacies" (p. 136). In other words, therapists become trusted, private, real people (i.e., friends) who provide guidance in the struggle for self-understanding. Other writings acknowledge the nontransferential ways in which a therapist's gender, age, humor, style, and physical features affect patients (Tyson, 1980). No doubt my gender, age, and easy fit with Carla furthered the positive aspects in our real relationship.

In contrast to the uncovering inherent in psychoanalysis, the emphasis in supportive psychotherapy is not on the past, but rather on the here-and-now. In analysis and insight-oriented uncovering psychotherapy, the primary focus is on inner conflicts; reconstructions of the past; and reexperiencing through examination of feelings, displacements, and the transference observed in the treatment situation. Overall, the focus of supportive psychotherapy is on current ego functioning, current object relationships, and regulations of self-esteem, via receipt of empathic support, acceptance, soothing, and admiration from a discreet, trusted person who clearly demonstrates warmth, affection, and respect. Self psychology offers the most sweeping supportive alterations of classic analytic stance and goals in the treatment process. Kohut (1984) stated that self psychologists commonly work in what he viewed as a more easygoing, relaxed, emotionally available fashion. Though not claiming that this greater relaxation is the sole province of self psychology, Kohut did believe that this approach permits greater emotional availability and spontaneity by the therapist, with a resultant "generally calmer and friendlier atmosphere" based on the expanded scope of empathy. Self psychology is not offering a new kind of empathy; rather, informed by new theory, "the self psychologist can empathically perceive configurations that would otherwise have escaped his notice" (Kohut, 1984, p. 84). These, I believe, include cross-cultural and cross-racial values, goals, and belief systems.

CASE OF CARLA, CONTINUED: EXAMPLE OF THE REAL RELATIONSHIP IN THE TREATMENT OF AN AMERICAN-BORN HISPANIC WOMAN

The real relationship in the treatment of Carla was characterized by the above-noted warmth and respect. Some self-disclosure was provided, and I never withheld reasons for schedule changes, or direct answers to numerous appropriate questions. Carla often brought in and shared her journal entries, papers she was working on in graduate school, positive evaluations she had received at work, and so forth. I deliberately chose not to reject or analyze these offerings, nor did I withhold genuine admiration and respect for Carla's productions. The more classic neutral therapeutic stance was scrupulously avoided, and Carla was able to utilize a range of supportive interventions, as well as interpretations and other interventions typical of insight-oriented psychotherapy.

Active discussions focused on Carla's long-standing eating disturbance, which resulted in our exploring together what Palombo

(1985) calls "the nature of the [individual's] experience" without making distant generalizations about the intrapsychic states" based on the symptoms. Carla, like many patients with bulimia, continued for some time to binge and purge at times of stress, but was helped to figure out why she did so. After several years of therapy, she no longer purged by vomiting. For more than 1½ years now, she has been free of the binge–purge cycle. Her excellent level of control began when she became pregnant. She became highly motivated to maintain her own and her unborn child's health, and with my guidance was able to eat wisely and appropriately. Previously, she could not consistently use the help available regarding limits and food regulation. Now she has been able to sustain her new nutritious regimen throughout the pregnancy and several months of nursing. Her postdelivery weight is ideal and has been comfortably maintained.

As Carla developed empathy for herself, modeled on my empathy for her, she became more self-accepting. She could manage sexual expression, aggression, anxiety, and food with increasing ease. She now speaks of having such a sense of mastery that she'd never collapse in panic. Her empathy for herself is reflected in better self-esteem, which, as noted earlier, has come to include more positive feelings about her cultural identity. Her proficiency with Spanish had diminished, because she had avoided speaking Spanish except when visiting her parents. This all changed during the second half of her therapy, whereby she came to have a sense of pride in her ethnic and cultural heritage. She regained her fluency with her first language via a commitment to working with Hispanic clients. Her pleasure at her bilingual fluency was striking, as was her growing pleasure in learning more about both Mexico and Ecuador, her parents' birthplaces.

Carla believes that, and often discusses and describes how, treatment enabled her to reach a racial/cultural level of comfort—that is, a stage of "integrated awareness" (Atkinson et al., 1998; Sue & Sue, 1999). Patients at this advanced stage "have acquired an inner sense of security as their self-identity. They have pride in their racial/cultural heritage yet can exercise a desired level of personal freedom and autonomy. Other cultures and races are appreciated, and there is a development towards becoming more multi-cultural in perspective" (Sue & Sue, 1999, p. 141).

Carla's development of empathy for herself illustrates "one of the most important contributions of self psychology to the therapeutic work with individuals with eating disorders. From this perspective, a major goal of therapy is helping people recognize who they are, and to accept themselves fully, with all of their own characteristics[, both] 'good' and 'bad' " (Barth, 1991, p. 241). For Carla, these characteristics include her femininity, body image, value system, professional identity, and newly gained cultural identity.

DISCUSSION OF ETHNIC/CULTURAL ISSUES IN THE REAL RELATIONSHIP WITH CARLA

Moving beyond a traditional intrapsychic focus, psychoanalytic theory has broadened its lens to include relational issues (object relations theory) and self-esteem (self psychology). Likewise, in the process of attempting to provide responsive cross-cultural psychotherapy, it is necessary for a clinician to be sensitive to a patient's cultural identity development. It is essential that therapists recognize differences among members of the same minority group with respect to their cultural identity. Cultural identity models with stages of development must be used flexibly, with a recognition that "cultural identity development is a dynamic process, not a static one" (Sue & Sue, 1999, p. 141).

When Carla began to work with me, she was not only self-depreciating, but depreciating of her Hispanic group membership. She was overly appreciating of white Midwest society in general, as well as of the powerful Jewish community in the community where she grew up (as described earlier). She felt very much the outsider and exception until she went east to a large urban city for college, and then moved to New York City for subsequent residence and employment. The greater diversity and cosmopolitan nature of these urban settings gave her a measure of anonymity and comfort. She has often found it amazing and paradoxical that she discovered herself and her cultural pride in her treatment with a white Jewish therapist, who, she believes, respected her Hispanic culture more than she herself originally did. Thus Carla's attachment to me, her therapist, was not based on race, but on our ability to share, understand, and accept our world views. "In other words, attitudinal similarity between therapist and client is a more important dimension than membership group similarity" (Sue & Sue, 1999, p. 141). Although the various models regarding cultural identity do not take into account class, age, or gender, Carla demonstrated and spoke of her sense that my awareness of my own cultural values and hers (including her world view), as well as our client–therapist fit, seemed based on our ability to send and receive both verbal and nonverbal messages, and thereby to intimately understand each other.

Sue and Sue (1999) describe *personalismo* as a basic cultural value of Hispanic Americans. Once trust has been established, a Hispanic client may develop a close personal bond with his or her therapist. The therapist may be viewed as a friend and given gifts. These behaviors should not be taken as evidence of dependency or an absence of boundaries. Thus warm acceptance accompanied some nontraditional exchange of gifts—flowers and other tokens of regard, concern, or achievement. For example, when I was seriously ill and hospitalized, I received a note and flowers from Carla; similarly, I sent small gifts to her upon her graduation from her master's degree program, when she married, and when she gave birth to her child.

Carla's real-life major achievements—namely, acquiring graduate training, entering a profession that delights and pleases her, making a solid and healthy marriage, and giving birth to a child—are most significant, and all seem to be based in her successful resolution of her Latina/Hispanic American identity. Her acceptance and pride in her culture and ethnicity are underscored by her better relationships with her family of origin, her improved self-esteem, and her sense that positive ethnic identity represents a successful outcome of her therapy.

CHAPTER SIX

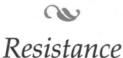

Resistance

RESISTANCE DEFINED AND DESCRIBED

Resistance in psychotherapy is universal, as all individuals and families instinctively resist change in the status quo. "Resistance" includes all patterns of feelings and behaviors that operate to prevent change. These oppositional patterns may be conscious or unconscious; deliberate or inadvertent; and manifested by a whole family, by one of its members, or even by the therapist him- or herself.

Resistance is dealt with from the onset of contact, and more intensively during the middle phase of therapy, following the assessment and the selection of the appropriate intervention (which includes determination of the frequency of contact).

Being in the business of bringing about change, therapists encounter resistance continually. However great the distress people feel, they resist asking for help, and having asked for help, they resist being influenced by the professional they have employed to help them. This resistance may be expressed overtly, through missed appointments, or blatant refusals to comply with the terms of the therapeutic contract;

but more frequently it is expressed covertly . . . [via] an apparent inability to understand the therapist's comments, or pervasive and persistent refusals to give up old expectations or behaviors. On the surface, resistance in psychotherapy would appear to be an irrational process which serves no useful purpose. Yet, irrational as it may seem, resistance is universal. (Anderson & Stewart, 1983, p. 1)

Despite therapists' expectations of resistance, it can feel personal, causing them to become frustrated, insecure, or even actively rejecting of their patients. Young practitioners may regard the struggle as due to their lack of experience; experienced therapists can find ongoing resistance wearing and draining, resulting in a sense of burnout and/or a loss of creative energy.

Resistance should be distinguished from a lack of motivation for change, or a lack of interest in entering therapy and forming a relationship with a professional person. Some types of resistance are present from the beginning of treatment and are characteristic of a patient's emotional structure; these forms are called "character resistance." Character resistance is distinguished from the opposition that arises in the course of therapy, to defend internal conflict. Regardless of its origins, resistance should not be viewed pejoratively, as it operates through the ego and demonstrates ego development. A total lack of defenses and resistance is an ominous sign, suggesting lack of psychic structure, decompensation, or a propensity to merge and comply indiscriminately. It is important to understand what the patient is avoiding and why. Therefore, resistance should not be assaulted with confrontation or intellectualized reflections and interpretations. This injunction corresponds with the self-psychological view of defense and resistance, whereby the self is seen as protecting itself not from the alarming emergence of dangerous drives and wishes, but rather from the possible repetition of significant psychological injury, especially traumatic assaults on self-esteem that occurred in childhood. Resistance is thus seen as safeguarding what remains of a healthy self (Kohut, 1984).

Freud (1900/1952), the first to recognize resistance, discovered that patients rejected his interpretations; he came to view resistance, like defenses, as a protective reflex against the intense anxiety inherent in facing unacceptable feelings, wishes, thoughts, and impulses. Freud initially considered resistance to be a conscious and intentional withholding of information because of distrust of the analyst, shame, fear of rejection, or the like. In his early work, Freud discovered that patients could not maintain free associations and sooner or later failed to mention something that occurred to them. Tardiness, overt attempts to win the analyst's approval, and engaging in a battle of wits were viewed as typically surrendered in the face of the analysts's exhortations. Unconscious resistance posed greater problems and commonly occurred throughout the course of therapy as an avoidance of discussing significant data.

Early psychoanalytic techniques, derived from structural theory, designated three types of resistance: resistance of the id, of the ego, and of the superego. Resistance emanating from the id is apparent in the patient's unwillingness to give up pleasure, no matter what price is paid internally; resistance of the ego is manifested in the appearance and tenacious use of unconscious defense mechanisms of the ego (which continue despite efforts to explore and analyze them); superego resistance is apparent in the persistence of guilt feelings and the need of punishment, and in negative therapeutic reactions (to guard against pleasure and success). Freud (1926) later subdivided ego resistance into three subtypes: repressive resistance and subsequent repetition compulsion; transference resistance; and resistance due to secondary gain (i.e., the hidden benefits of sustaining symptomatology). Classic theory dictates interpretation of resistance; more contemporary theorists posit other approaches, citing the limitations of interpretations.

Resistance typically continues to appear, even when repeated and accurate interpretations are offered. The only method with which to counter resistance is "working through," which is most thoroughly and affectively achieved via analysis (i.e., intensive, uncovering treatment). (See Chapter 8 for a fuller discussion of working through.) To minimize resistance, Freud devised many cornerstone analytic techniques. The couch, for example, enables a patient to direct his or her perceptions inward rather than engage in a more active interpersonal exchange with the analyst. The couch generally gives the patient more freedom to fantasize, free-associate, and develop transference feelings toward the analyst. The frequency of sessions stimulates continuity of the flow of material and helps maintain a focus on the treatment relationship. More contemporary treatment models, such as self psychology and intersubjectivity analytic technique, caution that resistance should not be assaulted with confrontation or intellectualized reflections and interpretations (as I have stated above). By contrast, those clinicians conducting short-term dynamic psychotherapy advocate active and direct confrontation from the very beginning of treatment (Davanloo, 1980; see especially Malan, 1980), and recommend that resistance be dealt with relentlessly.

Resistance is not a phenomena restricted to patients; in fact, it can be produced by helping systems and by (and in) therapists themselves. Anderson and Stewart (1983) note the rigidity of many institutional and administrative systems and the resistance of therapists, which can interfere with engaging clients and supporting the ongoing work of treatment. Institutions can be wedded to old attitudes and practices that interfere with engaging clients and/or interfere with needed outreach. Clinicians can be resistive due to competence anxiety, "therapist fatigue," and burnout.

ETHNIC/CULTURAL FACTORS THAT CAN OPERATE IN RESISTANCE

When a clinician is working with a culturally different client, the clinician's cultural countertransference can be a major source of resistance and can disrupt the treatment process, or even interfere with engaging the client. As described in Chapter 1, the multidisciplinary mental health field as a whole has come to the disturbing realization that therapeutic services for ethnically diverse groups lack effectiveness (Abramovitz & Murray, 1983; Atkinson, 1985; Sue, 1988; Sue

& Sue, 1990). As noted in Chapter 1, Perez Foster (1998a) reminds us that despite earlier warnings and injunctions, stereotypes and racist attitudes about the presumed inability of immigrants and clients of color to use insight-oriented theories continue. Refusal to accept such clients' capacity for self-observation and insight is not only a gross example of clinician resistance, but a "dangerous bias" (Perez Foster, 1998a). Perez Foster also mentions the "therapist's own feelings of sadness, despondency, or guilt about the client's life circumstances, or therapist reactions that include confusion [and] fears of prejudice towards an ethnic stranger" (p. 255). Clients commonly recognize these attitudes at varying levels of consciousness. This can propel a culturally different client to sustain resistances, and in particular to "completely endorse minority-held views and to reject the dominant values of society and culture" (Sue & Sue, 1999, p. 133).

It is not always possible to supply patients with therapists who match them on all cultural characteristics, such as class, color, race, and religion. "Furthermore, such cultural similarities are not always an advantage. As any anthropologist knows, it is far more difficult to study one's own culture than a foreign one, because too many things are taken for granted and too many blind spots are likely to coincide" (Anderson & Stewart, 1983, p. 141). Therapists in unmatched therapeutic dyads must be aware of their own cultural values and norms, and should make every effort not to impose these on their patients; rather, the patients must be helped to make clear what *their* values and customs are. A lack of knowledge, combined with a spirit of inquiry, can be an asset. It can facilitate dialogue and sharing of expectations, beliefs, and customs, and can demonstrate a therapist's willingness to learn about and to respect a patient's perspective.

As noted in Chapter 4, the therapeutic alliance cannot be taken for granted; it must be painstakingly built by the efforts of both patient and therapist. Herman (1992) notes that traumatic experiences frequently damage a client's ability to enter into a trusting relationship and form an alliance. Thus the therapist can expect difficulties in forming a working alliance if the patient has suffered severe traumas, particularly within the context of family relationships.

CASE OF SOPHIA: EXAMPLE OF RESISTANCE IN THE TREATMENT OF A EUROPEAN-BORN ITALIAN WOMAN

Development, Family, and Psychosocial History

Sophia had been seen in therapy once before, and several years later sought therapy with me. She has been in treatment with me for close to 2 years, taking an "intermission" over one summer following her exhaustion after her mother had a heart attack—a health crisis that required much time and support. She resumed therapy with me, seeing it as a source of assistance and relief, because of feeling consistently misunderstood (Basch, 1980). Her presenting complaints centered on her ambivalence and fears about her future, related to her lengthy separation from her husband and her prolonged hesitation to finalize their divorce. Because she had married her high school boyfriend, she felt extremely unexperienced and shy about the prospect of meeting new men, dating, and surviving the "singles" world. She had never been involved with another man before her husband; although she was certain that she and her husband could not improve their relationship, she feared being alone and childless, and felt inept about moving on and making new friends.

Additional presenting concerns centered on what Sophia described as her "lack of discipline"—that is, her long standing patterns of procrastination, depression, and difficulty in awakening promptly and getting to work punctually. In addition, her problems with food management had created a recurrent cycle: overconsumption of junk food and weight gains of 10–15 pounds, followed by extraordinary dieting, successful weight loss, and a short-lived sense of improved self-esteem. Apparently, recurrent shame and depression would trigger the poor eating habits. Despite the realities of these problems, Sophia was (and remains) an extraordinarily beautiful woman, of average height and weight, a brunette with a wondrous complexion and facial features. Aged 32 when she began treatment with me, she has long functioned productively and successfully in a most demanding high-level position in a furniture manufacturing company. Her titles at work, salary, bonuses, and areas of responsibility have continually expanded. Her pleasure over her professional accomplishments has fluctuated, however, and often she resents the central role her job plays in what she describes as her "workaholic" existence.

Sophia has remained quite isolated socially; her primary social relationship is with one best friend at work. However, she is very close to her family of origin—namely, her widowed mother and two brothers, one of whom is married and has children she's attached to. She was also very close to her father, who died 7 years ago. Sophia feels she's made little progress in adequately separating from her mother, due to her being the only girl in an immigrant, traditional Italian family. As the only daughter, she was and still is the one who must bear primary responsibility for her mother. Our work together has revealed the continued resonance of her immigrant experience in childhood; she recalls being a shy, tongue-tied child, with no knowledge of English at first. As is the case in many immigrant groups, the children did learn English while the parents did not, thus requiring the children to act as interpreters and to manage money (e.g., checking accounts and bill paying) for their parents. Sophia recounts being cast into the role of the "parentified child" and having to provide much caretaking of her parents, particularly her mother. In addition, she had to assume much of the care for her siblings and the home, with cooking and cleaning responsibilities at a very young age.

Since separating from her husband several years ago, she has resided in an apartment beneath her mother's apartment, in a building her parents owned for many years and her mother continues to own. Sophia pays a low rent for what's always been a rental unit in this family-owned building. Like many Italian families, hers never chose to move, despite increased means that would allow for a better residence. Sophia hopes eventually to move out of her ethnic enclave (a neighborhood she's ashamed of), but sky-high rents continue to keep her where she is—a dilemma, she feels, because her residence further inhibits her social life. Despite yearning for a more cosmopolitan and interesting life, Sophia continues to hold back, never exploring the city and all its cultural, artistic, and social offerings.

Sophia has shared with me her struggles as she straddles two worlds (i.e., her old neighborhood, and her professional world and different identity in the city). She's described how she went to great lengths to transform her appearance and patterns of speech, moving out of the world of "Guidos" and "Guidoettes" (her derogatory terms for stereotyped Italian males and females, replete with gold chains and gold crosses, teased hair, and overdressing). She has related in detail the transformation she wrought, and the contrast between her current and past appearance, manner of speech, and personal style.

In her family, advanced education was not ignored, but was only mildly encouraged by her parents. Sophia and both brothers briefly attended college. Her brothers chose to join her father's construction company and to earn as much as possible as soon as possible. Sophia couldn't handle her social isolation as a commuter student, because her parents refused to let her move and live on campus. For Sophia, college was a lonely experience where she felt out of place, despite ease in handling her academic work, and so she abruptly withdrew. She has since had some vague thoughts of part-time attendance, but has not pursued this, having no special interests to pursue. She earns a six-figure salary, and is not held back by lack of a college degree at her job (her sole place of employment, where she began when she was an older teenager as a part-time stock girl).

According to Rotunno and McGoldrick (1982), Italian families view education and vocational training as secondary to security, affection, and family relationships. In contrast to other ethnic groups (e.g., Jews and Asians), whose members make enormous sacrifices for educating their children, college is not usually expected in Italian working-class families. Education often poses a threat to the family system: "Education meant that a young person would come under the influence of outside authorities and perhaps leave home to study" (Rotunno & McGoldrick, 1982, p. 344). Similar views have prevailed about work: "While middle-class Americans view the lack of interest in careers and professional advancement of Italian Americans as a deficiency in [their] characters, Italian Americans view the achievement oriented action of Americans as disgracefully selfish" (Papajohn & Spiegel, 1975, p. 109).

Sophia feels she's always been working since early childhood, when she had to help her mother with housecleaning, cooking, laundry, and the like. Her account of herself doing the dishes at age 7, standing on a chair to reach the sink, was very poignant; she shared her initial eagerness and enthusiasm, all of which declined over time, as the demands on her increased profoundly. Since she was 7 years old, inordinate amounts of housework were assigned to her. She was never free Saturdays to join friends, in contrast to her overindulged brothers, who in the true Italian cultural tradition were given no household responsibilities (she even had to clean up after them). She resented all of this, but did not refuse to work, even in college when she had to vacuum, dust, change linens, do laundry, iron, and wait on her brothers and father. "No one was officious or demanding; it was just the expectation of a traditional, old-world Italian family." In addition, her mother's neediness and major emotional problems inhibited any rebellion. Sophia's traditional Italian family adhered to well-worn patterns of role differentiation between sons and daughters:

> Sons are given much greater latitude prior to marriage. A bit of acting-out is expected, even subtly encouraged as a measure of manliness . . . girls . . . are more restricted than their brothers and boy cousins. They are given more guidance and supervision and, in particular, are taught to eschew personal achievements in favor of respect and service to their parents. (Rotunno & McGoldrick, 1982, p. 348)

Since Sophia's career success, her brothers have often approached her for sizable sums of money they want to "borrow," both for business and for their personal expenses. After a number of unpaid loans, she has curtailed lending or giving her earnings to them. Her major self-indulgences are lavish vacations to beaches in Mexico and the Caribbean with her close girlfriend. She also devotes some of her income to stylish, tasteful clothes and to her car, which is rarely more than 2 years old. She also saves a portion of her salary. This somewhat compensates for all the years that she describes supporting herself and her husband financially. He had worked with her brothers in their family-owned building/renovating business, where incomes chronically fluctuated. His lack of ambition and personal growth, in her opinion, caused their growing apart.

Sophia's mother suffers from long-standing major emotional problems, which have required one psychiatric hospitalization and continual usage of medications. Growing up, Sophia always felt ashamed of her mother, because of her vulnerabilities and lack of English. She would guiltily wish that she had another mother. She became more attached to her teachers and was always "teacher's pet"; this was particularly so with a high school teacher, who urged and supported her college attendance. She still maintains contact with this woman, who, in fact, was the one to recommend psycho- therapy originally.

In the course of our work together, Sophia has become less guilty and less impatient with her mother. In fact, she has been sur- prised that her mother has voiced some intelligent and wise views about her and about life in general. Her mother has always worked in a woman's hat factory, where she sews and embroiders. The mother is described as shy and lacking a circle of friends; she is more closely connected to family members and the church. Sophia de- scribes herself and her brothers as lapsed Catholics, with no atten- dance or contact with the church.

Sophia's mother has recently accepted her daughter's need for privacy and quiet time at the end of the work day, and so, does not rush to greet her daily upon her return home; in addition, she's de- scribed as more reasonable and understanding about Sophia's nu- merous vacations and business trips, and her hopes eventually to move away to an apartment in the city. Although Sophia's decision to divorce was not opposed by her family, her mother is described as most desirous to see her remarried and settled, with children and a family of her own. Meeting men was and remains a major problem. No one in the family knows single men to introduce her to, and she goes nowhere except for dinners in the city where she never encoun- ters single men. The bar scene repels her, and she participates in no sports, whereby she might meet other single people. Men met at work are commonly married or of no interest to her. Until very re- cently she'd go nowhere alone, and has lately felt a sense of pride that she actually went to a local beach alone, when her best friend wasn't available.

Cultural Identity for Sophia and Her Family

As the treatment alliance has deepened, Sophia has been able to share the details of her childhood—the pain and upheaval of the immigration experience, which she recognizes is still with her, causing shyness and inhibition. In her first therapy, the experience of migration and other ethnic/cultural factors were never touched on or explored. When she was 7 years old, the family moved from a small southern farming town near Naples, Italy, to Toronto, Canada, and 2 years later to the United States. Family members already located in Canada and the United States were supportive, taking them in until they could secure their own housing.

Not until high school did Sophia feel a part of any social group, since earlier she'd felt intimidated by peers. As a parentified child, she had to provide much help and support to her parents, and so had little time for friendships. Later she got involved with a fast crowd, whose members smoked, drank, cut classes, and generally were only interested in finding boyfriends or girlfriends. It was during this period of her adolescence that she connected with her one and only boyfriend, a very handsome, long-haired teen, with no ambitions or special abilities. They ultimately married when she was 24, and much of her focus was on making and saving money to buy and then maintain a house. They had no circle of friends, since her husband was indifferent to much beyond spending his own money and relying on her earnings. Sophia has described him as low-keyed and dependent on her and her older brothers and father, for whom he worked, showing little initiative in seeking more construction contracts or even in working very hard at the job.

At the end of the first year of our therapeutic work together, Sophia finalized her divorce, doing so without rancor or anger. In fact, Sophia eagerly desired to remain friends; so did her ex-husband until recently, when he began seeing an old high school friend, who was jealous and objected to any ongoing conversations and contacts with Sophia. Sophia has been saddened by this reality: "Passive as ever, he's accepted his new girlfriend's ultimatum, and it hurts to think we'll never see each other again, or never converse again." Her ex-husband no longer works for her brothers; he recently obtained training in building maintenance and repair, and now makes a better income than when he was married to Sophia. She claims to have no regrets, since basically, even with some improvement in his income, he's not grown or really changed. The increasing disparity between them regarding income, work status, ambition, and curiosity about life remains.

While Sophia has moved ahead, she feels somewhat adrift. Because she is more successful than people of her past, she feels somewhat estranged from them, and yet she is insufficiently connected to new people in her new life. Sophia feels the old shame, shyness, and tongue-tied inhibitions of her immigrant childhood (although, with the help of therapy, these have recently lessened). She experiences fewer bouts of sadness and real depression, despite recognizing that she feels caught on the horns of a bicultural dilemma—coming from a traditional, old-world, working-class Italian family, where she's broken the rules regarding gender roles. If her parents had become more Americanized, or if her brothers had become better educated, she believes the conflicts for her would have been less. Rotunno and McGoldrick (1982), and other authors they cite, suggest that Italian children have "more conflict about their upwardly mobile aspirations, which their families perceive as threatening" (p. 349). This contrasts with other ethnic groups such as Jews and WASPs, whose members fear not living up to their parents' expectations and ambitions. In keeping with Italian family mores and characteristics, Sophia is stressed by the fact that she earns as much as or more than her brothers, especially her older brother, who has a family to support. However, here too her sense of guilt and discomfort have lessened over the course of our work together.

Although Sophia's family of origin is described as proud of her work and economic success, she feels a strong undercurrent of ambivalence and resistance, which mirrors her own. She sees her level of acculturation as greater than that of her siblings, but suspects that it remains at a superficial level (i.e., the manifest level of dress, appearance, employment, and earnings), and not at the more latent, in-depth level, since her basic self-regard or self-esteem still falters and fluctuates, though the swings are now less extreme. It was not until we examined comparative salaries at her place of work that she could assert herself and take some initiative to request fairer salary compensation, equal to that of male executives with her level of responsibility. She recognized carrying into the work arena or "work family" the sociocultural Italian attitudes of her family of origin, in which males are more esteemed, and women work very hard with less compensation and recognition. Treatment has enabled her to be more assertive and self-assured, despite her continued resistance to trying new things socially.

Sophia has recently recognized her lack of interest or pride in her Italian heritage. She has felt little pleasure in her being bilingual, even when she was able to converse fluently while touring in Italy, on the few trips made with her family of origin. In her adult years, she has not visited Italy. She ruefully acknowledges no familiarity with Italian music, art, or literature. Because her dad occasionally listened to opera, she feels some affinity for this cultural activity, but has never attended a live performance. What has emerged is, instead, a sense of stigma and shame about her ethnic roots. She remains resistive to any new exposure or self-education about her ethnic culture.

Because of the demands at her job, including frequent long hours, Sophia has not had the time or made the time for any hobbies or interests (photography, a cooking class, tennis or golf lessons, etc.), all of which she's frequently thought of. In addition to her employment is her responsibility for her mother. She handles all of her mother's routines (e.g., medical and dental appointments), as well as providing some degree of companionship. Although her brothers are warm and connected to their mother, they do not accept any responsibility even for home repairs (which on occasion are badly needed, and which they can easily provide, since they are carpenters/builders with their own company). The recurrent situation used to enrage Sophia, but now she maintains relative calm, hires contractors (since her mother can afford to pay for the work), and informs her brothers of the paradox. Sophia has not surrendered responsibility for her mother, but she has given up her nagging, ranting stance with her brothers. Sophia finds her mother's "typically Italian" style of continued oversolicitousness for her brothers ironic, given their lack of concern/consideration for her. While their father was not "authoritative or rigid in role setting and guidelines for behavior" (Rotonno & McGoldrick, 1982, p. 349), Sophia doubts that her brothers would so procrastinate and/or neglect their mother's needs if he were still alive. In the last year or so, Sophia defines her family relationships as less conflictual and more enjoyable. She's feeling less angry with her mother and brothers, and closer to each of them.

Forms of Resistance Exhibited by Sophia

Sophia views her better relationships with her family as a positive outcome of her therapy. However, despite her gains in treatment, she remains steadfast in her refusal to increase the number of sessions per week; she persists in maintaining only one weekly session, for which she commonly arrives late, due to her refusal to allow sufficient time upon leaving work for commuting to her appointment. Her addiction to her "workaholic" existence constitutes what Freud noted as a form of "unconscious resistance," because it results in tardiness, as well as an avoidance of discussing significant data. In Sophia's case, these data include her social isolation, romantic longings, sexual fantasies, and struggles regarding femininity.

> [Addiction is defined] as a syndrome that occurs most commonly in women and consists of periods of depression, feelings of ugliness and over-eating or over-drinking, alternating with periods of normal or elated mood, feelings of beauty and aesthetic behavior. By psychoanalytic definition these patients show a pre-oedipal mother conflict with unconscious hatred of the mother and of femininity: Their urge to eat is an attempt to incorporate something to counteract femininity: milk, penis, child and/or narcissistic supplies which soothe anxieties. (Campbell, 1981, p. 13)

In treatment, Sophia feels safest talking about her professional life, work relationships, and professional aspirations. The workplace is where she invests her greatest energy, at the expense of her personal life. Whereas Freud stressed the abilities to work, love, and play as all needed for a balanced existence, Sophia remains primarily fixated on the issue of work, apparently because she fears further probing and perhaps better understanding her restricted approach to life. As the definition of "addiction" above suggests, she suffers from bouts of overeating, depression, and feeling ugly and unattractive, despite her actual physical beauty. Despite ample financial resources, she does not allow herself routine pleasures and indulgences such as participation in sports or membership in a health club, where socializing could occur. She does not attend any of the myriad of cultural, artistic, or entertainment activities that are available in the city. Resistance of the ego is apparent in her use of ego defenses of rationalization, denial, and avoidance; superego resistance is apparent in her need for punishment (i.e., overwork) and in the persistence of guilt feelings that preclude and guard against pleasure.

DISCUSSION OF ETHNIC/CULTURAL ISSUES IN SOPHIA'S TREATMENT AND RESISTANCE

Like Perlmutter (1996), I prefer the term "culturally responsive" to similar terms, such as "culturally competent." Perlmutter notes that other authors (Pedersen & Ivey, 1993; Vargas & Koss-Chioino, 1992) also emphasize responsiveness in practice ability, and particularly in the capacity to "manage cultural complexity and respond appropriately to dynamic changes in cultural salience" (Perlmutter, 1996, p. 13). The concept of "responsiveness" also corresponds with some of the newer conceptions in psychoanalytic theory, in self psychology, and in the intersubjectivity theory—most clearly articulated by Bacal (1998a, 1998b) and Stolorow, Atwood, and Brandchaft (1994)—that I believe I have fruitfully drawn on in my work with Sophia. (See below for a more detailed discussion of these.)

Whereas many researchers/clinicians describe Italian families and Italian clients as restricted and slow to offer acceptance to an outsider, this has not been the case with Sophia. She had a comfortable prior experience with a non-Italian therapist, as well as positive connections with others outside the family system, given her long-standing close ties with her former teachers and present employers. Moreover, Sophia does not demonstrate what is considered by some researchers and clinicians as an Italian penchant for histrionics. Rather, she has silently endured a lifelong hunger for maternal nurturance. When the family immigrated from Italy, she lost a substantial amount of maternal parenting, due to her mother's full-time employment in Toronto and New York City. In addition, the mother's emotional vulnerabilities and lack of English created role reversal, whereby Sophia had to assume parenting functions—helping her mother, often caring for her mother, and serving as her mother's interpreter. At a very young age, as described earlier, she had to handle payment of bills and the like. Her overly close connection to teachers since grade school was, in her view, a search for mothering; specifically, she was seeking a connection with a maternal admirable object she could lean on and learn from, as opposed to one she'd have to teach, care for, and be ashamed of. In therapy, she has made a quick attachment to maternal objects, who have become in fact idealized objects, much as her teachers were in childhood.

Although Sophia's family settled in a predominantly Italian community near relatives, the family has not interfered with her employment outside the community. College outside of the community was also accepted but residence at home was expected and adhered to by Sophia. Thus, since high school, she has moved in two worlds: that of her family and the Italian community, and that of the mainstream American community. At times Sophia feels as though she has a false sense of identity, as she attempts to adapt to and fit into the wider community. It has been crucial in therapy with Sophia to be sensitive to this reality, and not to push for independence and individuality. Her level of family enmeshment has not provided Sophia what she considers as supports; rather, it puts inordinate demands on her that cannot be criticized and/or disrupted, given her need for maintenance of her close family ties. I believe that slow, gentle, empathic reflections, rather than expressions of advice or of an implied preference for separation, have been and remain the indicated interventions.

Responsive cross-cultural treatment requires that the clinician develop a therapeutic "third eye" or "third ear" (cf. Reik, 1949) for sensing the presence of minimal cues to sociocultural patterns, as well as for detecting "partially hidden signs of individual uniqueness" (Fish, 1996, p. 133). It is crucial that the therapist not attempt to influence the client directly or indirectly or to challenge resistance in a manner that will cause the client to change his or her values in the direction of the therapist's particular values. Fish (1996) emphasizes professional ethics in stressing this sort of restraint; he additionally notes that attempts to change clients' values can backfire, undermine progress in treatment, or even lead to the abrupt termination of treatment. It is for these reasons (among others) that I, like Fish, have advocated a strategy of supporting the client's values in ways that can make the attainment of therapeutic goals more likely. Thus, in Sophia's therapy, I have taken care not to emphasize my own preferences and values—for example, separation/individuation, feminism, higher education, romantic attachments, a richer and wider social network, and career ambitions that might risk alienation from the family. Cultural relativism is of immense value in working with patients from a different sociocultural background. Fish states that "sociocultural awareness is quite like the sociological concept of class consciousness, except that it is an awareness relating to membership in virtually any group with similar backgrounds or in similar situations, and not just an economic class" (p. 129).

THE CLINICIAN'S ETHNIC/CULTURAL HERITAGE: ITS ROLE IN SOPHIA'S TREATMENT

As I have discussed in Chapter 2, the researchers and writers examining therapy with culturally diverse individuals all emphasize that "clinicians need to be aware of their own cultural identity and their attitudes and beliefs towards ethnic minorities, because these will affect their relationships with patients" (Lu et al., 1995, p. 477). Pinderhughes (1982, 1989) and others recommend that clinicians explore their own ethnic background by considering its historic influence on their attitudes, feelings, and behaviors. Pinderhughes recommends self-questions about one's feelings about belonging to one's ethnic group, one's positive and negative feelings about one's ethnic identity, one's recognition of the values of one's ethnic group, and one's experience as a person having or lacking power in relation to ethnic identity, class identity, sexual identity, and professional identity. Thus I make the following (atypical) self-disclosures in this section, which have not been shared with Sophia.

In contrast to Sophia—born in Europe, and a childhood immigrant twice, from Italy to Toronto and then from Toronto to New York City—I was born in the United States. My mother was also American-born, and was the middle child of Russian Jewish immigrants. They conformed to the Jewish stereotype of inordinate sacrifice for their children's educational advancement; however, my maternal grandparents demonstrated atypical emphasis on securing "equal opportunity" for their male and female children, all of whom obtained graduate school training. Despite my maternal grandfather's arriving penniless, years ahead of his wife (whom he later brought over), my maternal grandparents worked together and fared well economically, slowly and steadily improving their finances via sound real estate investments of a modest and secure sort. My maternal grandfather was an educated youth who had been considered a scholar in his village in Russia. In contrast, my grandmother was less well educated, since she had worked since childhood in a family-owned clothing shop. Her mother had died at the time of her birth, so she literally had no childhood, but had always worked as the "little woman" of the household.

My father was born in Russia; his family fled, from pogroms against Jews, but could only obtain entry into Canada. My paternal grandparents were working-class; my grandfather was a carpenter, who managed to obtain sufficient work that he could eventually provide a middle-class existence for his family, complete with home ownership and purchase of another residence used as rental-income-generating property. My father was the only child in his family who sought a college education, followed by professional training as a doctor. Upon graduation he sought an internship, which was all but unavailable to Jews in Montreal at that time, despite his very high standing in his medical school class. Thus he and his peers applied for training in the United States, crossing the Great Lakes into such American cities as Detroit, Cleveland, and Buffalo—cities with Jewish hospitals that would accept them. Thus, like Sophia, I too had a "Canadian" connection in my family, though it was of a vastly different nature from hers.

In my work with Sophia, I am conscious of her connection to my ethnic Jewish group—a minority population with an ethnic enclave in close proximity to her Italian neighborhoods in both Canada and the United States. Her later exposure to Jewish people was with some peers at school, many of her teachers, some physicians seen by family members, and her employers (the owners of the company where she's worked since late adolescence). My lifelong exposure to Italians has been with American-born Italians—some friends in lower school and high school, and others in later years, who were and are professional colleagues. My adult life contact with Italians has been with well-educated individuals—people with strong and sophisticated interests in the arts, as well as greater ethnic comfort and pride than demonstrated by my patient. Other Italian clients I've treated, in contrast to Sophia, have likewise been American-born and well-educated professionals.

Unlike my patient, but like my secure Italian friends, I grew up with a sense of confidence and pride in my ethnic heritage. Despite having suffered from being Jewish, both my parents and their families of origin were secure in and proud of their Jewish identity. The Orthodox religious practices of my grandparents were surrendered in my parents' home, but membership in a temple, activity in the Jewish community, and joyful celebration of holidays and traditions have characterized my lifelong experience. All family members in my nuclear and extended family exude a positive and very strong sense of Jewish identity. This security in our ethnic identity was further bolstered by pride in feminism and family wide higher education for males and females. My sibling and I, and almost all of our cousins, have graduate school training; professions as physicians, educators, or creative artists; high job satisfaction; and upper-middle-class incomes. These realities provide me, my family, and my extended family with a sense of having power, in striking contrast to my patient, who grew up feeling powerless. Sophia continues to feel some degree of helplessness and powerlessness and a generalized sense of shame, but this seems to be diminishing as her therapy supports her gaining better self-esteem and slowly but surely becoming assertive and self-protective. Her sense of pleasure in her work is still less than she'd like, but such is the nature of her tasks and of the politics at her company.

Sophia and her family were legal immigrants who arrived via the usual channels, originally from Italy, and then from Canada. In contrast, my family's immigrant experience (especially on my father's side) was as refugees—that is, persons who were forced to leave their country of origin (Russia) under political, economic, and social duress, and who voluntarily sought refuge in another country (Lum, 2000). My father actually became a refugee twice: in very early childhood when fleeing Russia, and later in life when he had to leave Canada for further medical training (thus experiencing economic and social, if not political, duress).

The emphasis on family solidarity is shared by Italian and Jewish families, as is the not uncommon practice of settling into neighborhoods of a distinctly ethnic character, especially upon arrival in North America. Maintenance of the original language of childhood is common in both groups, especially for first- and second-generation immigrants. It's frequently lost by the third generation, as was the case in our family.

I believe that my work with Sophia has been culturally responsive, because I have utilized my self-awareness about my own cultural context (Devore & Schlesinger, 1991; Sue & Sue, 1990), and because I have paid "simultaneous attention to [my patient's] individual and systemic concerns" (Devore & Schlesinger, 1991, p. 180).

SELF-PSYCHOLOGICAL AND INTERSUBJECTIVE PERSPECTIVES ON THE WORK WITH SOPHIA

Self-Psychological Perspectives

Narcissistic vulnerability commonly arises because early relationships were unstable, or because a caretaker's response was inadequate to meet the needs of a developing child. Kohut (1971) found that the diagnosis of a disorder of the self could best be made through careful observation of a narcissistic transference. For example, "That is when the analyst is perceived as an idealized source of soothing, loving affirmation and approval or a perfect other who is capable of solving all problems" (Solomon, 1991, p. 120). Often after only a few sessions in individual psychotherapy, such a narcissistic transference is easily discernible, as was the case in my early work with Sophia. As noted earlier, she's had a small number of significant and intense nonfamily attachments (i.e., one specific high school teacher she still has contact with, two therapists, and her closest girlfriend), whose presence seemingly helps her maintain a sense of cohesiveness. In work with depressed patients, Kohut stressed the importance of permitting selfobject transferences to emerge, to provide opportunities for "reparative/restorative interactions between therapist and patient" (Deitz, 1991, p. 196).

The self-psychological approach with depressed patients differs greatly from those of traditional drive theory and ego psychology, which emphasize mobilizing the patient's rage and encouraging its expression. When concepts of self-representation and selfobject transferences are utilized, the goal is to soothe—to achieve better regulation of mood and self-esteem. The clinician's soothing is accompanied by pacification, and by exploration without censure of "the protective functions of . . . social isolation[; this] demonstrates that he is in tune with the patient's disintegration anxiety and shame, concerning his precariously established self" (Kohut & Wolf, 1978, p. 424). It appears that my use of empathy in Sophia's case, as emphasized by self psychology, facilitated "perceptions of configurations that otherwise have escaped notice" (Kohut, 1984, p. 84). In fact, Sophia's childhood upheaval and her experience of the shame and pain of immigration were never considered in her original course of therapy. The current treatment process is best described as based on both self psychology and the theory of intersubjectivity (see below), which have informed my utilization of specific techniques of understanding, explanation, and interpretation. From the onset I attempted (seemingly successfully) to immerse myself empathically, thereby gaining a deeper emotional understanding of Sophia's demands, hopes, ambitions, struggles, resistances, and symptomatic behavior. Interpretations have been offered by way of providing explanations of the apparent dynamics and origins of Sophia's actions, behaviors, and transference manifestations. "The effect of understanding, interpreting and explaining have enhanced cognitive insight but this is secondary to the self psychology goal of providing structure building in consequence of optimal frustration" (Mishne, 1993, p. 309).

In keeping with this perspective, Sophia and I address current issues and functioning, and while maintaining interest in her past, we are continually attempting to examine "what forces are at work now that keep [Sophia] from activating aspects of the self that would allow [her] to feel better?" (Deitz, 1991, p. 197). Because her shame has been so pervasive, and has been presented overtly, we can identify and delineate Sophia's particular shame experiences. I have been able to convey my interest, empathy, and acceptance of this affect state, and to work with Sophia on the precipitants and manifestations of her lifelong sense of shame, in numerous areas in her life (Morrison, 1989). She has noted gradual and consistent relief, lessened depression, and better self-esteem.

Optimal Responsiveness and Other Intersubjective Concepts

"Optimal responsiveness," as explicated by Bacal (1998a, 1998b), describes both the clinician's therapeutic function and the patient's therapeutic experience as a result of an increasing awareness of the interactional/relational nature of the psychoanalytic process. In Bacal's conception, the therapist communicates with the patient in ways that "that particular patient experiences as usable for the cohesion, strengthening and growth of his self" (Bacal, 1998b, p. 142). Additionally noted is the way in which the clinician's response facilitates therapeutic relatedness, understood as a corrective selfobject relationship and experiences within an interactive reciprocal system. The therapist cannot expect or aim for perfection, but should simply be "himself or herself in the best way that he or she can, in order to enable the patient to use him or her therapeutically" (Bacal, 1998b, p. 167).

Optimal responsiveness entails the utilization of affect attunement to apprehend and understand the patient's subjective experiences, and this takes place in a relational or interactional system. Kohut (1984) spoke of "self–selfobject relationships," and Modell (1984) referred to a "two-person psychology." Mitchell (1988) described the "relational matrix," and Beebe and Lachmann (1988a, 1988b) labeled the treatment dyadic system a "mutual influential structure." Atwood and Stolorow (1984) first utilized the term "intersubjective context" to describe the treatment process, shaped by the "continually shifting psychological field cast by the interplay between the differently organized subjective worlds of patient and [therapist]" (Stolorow et al., 1994, p. 28).

The use of cultural responsiveness in clinical practice is suggested as an additional enriching element that further defines facets of the relational matrix or the intersubjective context. The clinician's observational stance is a two-person approach from within rather than outside the patient, and introspection and empathy are therefore essential. Years earlier, Schwaber (1979) offered some concepts that anticipated the intersubjective perspective. She stressed the differences between observing from inside and observing from outside the patient's state of mind, and between a focus on the patient's subjective inner reality and an attempt at objectivity. Cultural, ethnic, racial, and gender variables, which are all too often ignored, are inherent facets of a patient's selfobject configuration and subjective inner realities. Aspects of cultural and ethnic/racial identity are intrinsic to subjective experiences and must be included in efforts to offer what Kohut (1984, p. 78) and other self psychologists describe as the "corrective emotional experience," and what intersubjectivity theorists describe as the essence of cure—namely, attaining new principles of organizing experience (Stolorow & Atwood, 1992). "An intersubjective orientation 'requires' a continuous appreciation of the over-riding importance of the interplay of the subjective lives of both participants in the therapeutic situation" (Nattusa & Friedman, 1995, p. xiii).

Sensitivity to racial, ethnic, and cultural diversity is, I believe, enriched by both self psychology and intersubjectivity and likewise, they are enhanced when integrated with cultural responsiveness. I believe that this combination has sustained Sophia's involvement in treatment, despite her slow progress, her resistance, and her continued inhibitions (both socially and educationally). She remains fearful of and resistive to trying new leisure-time activities and new social experiences, and thereby continues to be rather socially isolated. Although I often ache for her continued somewhat lonely personal life, devoid of a wider circle of friends and the romantic partner she says she hopes for, I continue to accept her adherence to her position as an "old-world good Italian devoted daughter." I am certain that a more aggressive confrontation of her resistance, as recommended by various therapists conducting short-term psychotherapy (Davanloo, 1980, and especially Malan, 1980; Mann, 1973; Sifneos, 1973), would cause her to take flight and abruptly conclude treatment. "Clearly, in the psychoanalytic approach to treatment, resistance is not something to be overcome to get to the 'real' issues of therapy, since working through resistance *is* the therapy" (Anderson & Stewart, 1983, p. 5). Similarly, a self psychologist views forms of resistance as safeguarding what remains of a healthy self, and ordinarily does not "draw the patient's cognitive attention to them but rather tacitly conveys his understanding of his patient's current need to retain them' " (Bacal, 1990, pp. 262–263).

Therapy is a collaborative process that requires the client and the therapist to cooperate as partners in the therapeutic enterprise, and it is this alliance that is the central and enduring basis of the client's relationship to the therapist (Perlman, 1997). With Sophia, this has required accepting the wise words of Dostoyevsky: "Taking a new step, uttering a new word is what people fear the most." Thus I accept her fears and resistance, and as we both come to understand them better, they are slowly diminishing. Our continuing exploration of the resonance of the immigrant experience of her childhood is a key factor in this process.

CHAPTER SEVEN

Fixation, Regression, and Defenses

FIXATION

In considering "fixation" (a point of arrest)—that which holds children, adolescents, and adults back in the developmental scale, rendering them vulnerable, or incapable of assuming and/or mastering the normal tasks and roles commensurate with their chronological age—we note the tendency in psychic development for residual aspects of earlier phases to acquire and retain strong "charges" of psychic energy and to play a significant role in later development of mental functioning. Arrests of development can occur in instinctual, superego, and ego organization, permitting (in various degrees) the persistence of primitive ways of gaining satisfaction, of relating to people, and of reacting defensively to old or even outmoded dangers. In addition to insufficiently understood constitutional reasons for fixation (e.g., inherent differences in the functioning of various erogenous zones and in ego givens), there are inevitable experiences in which the developing, immature ego is overwhelmed by too much stress (A. Freud, 1977; Nagera, 1964). These traumatic experiences usually involve an unfortunate combination of excessive gratification and excessive frustration. For example, a bereaved young mother, suffering from her spouse's untimely death, allows their 3-year-old son to sleep with her; thus the child suffers not only the pain and frustration due to the loss of the father, but excessive gratification from inordinate closeness to and overstimulation from the mother. With disturbances of development and conflict over current functioning, regression or a falling back to earlier behavior and functioning occurs. Thus this boy, arrested and too tied to his mother, may seek overindulgence and inappropriate closeness with the mother when he is facing adolescent stressors. With disturbances of development and conflict over current functioning, regression to remnants of earlier functioning that are fixed in the psyche is possible, probable, and often unavoidable. Thus fixation generally implies pathology; syndromes or disorders are signs of fixation points to earlier trauma.

REGRESSION

"Regression" is the act of returning to earlier modes or levels of adaptation, or to points of fixation, in early trauma and arrest.

> Following the designation of Freud, [these modes or levels] are: 1) intrauterine; 2) infancy (early and late, extending from birth to approximately the fifth year; this period includes, among other things, the phases or oral, anal and genital organization); 3) latency (extending from about the age of five to puberty); 4) puberty (beginning at the onset of manhood or womanhood and continuing for two or three years; one of its main attributes is adult sexuality); 5) adolescence (beginning in the early or middle teens, its principal characteristics revolve around the reality principle, heterosexuality and sublimated interest); 6) adulthood (extending from the termination of the adolescent period to senescence); 7) climacterium; 8) senescence (the phase of decadence). (Campbell, 1981, p. 542)

There are two types of regression: "libidinal" and "ego" regression. Libidinal regression is a retreat to an earlier phase of instinctual organization, especially of the infantile period. Such a falling back occurs when a predetermined maturational step presents patients with difficulties they are unable to master. Often this is determined by earlier unresolved conflicts and anxieties, which leave areas of weakness in the preceding developmental phases (i.e., fixations), to which patients are more likely to regress. A simple example of libidinal regression may be observed when, at times of emotional stress, a bright 8-year-old child resumes thumb sucking (a habit previously abandoned). Aggression and aggressive moods are grouped under the category of libidinal drive expression. In childhood, the development of sexual drives is still fluid, and libidinal regression is common when a child is under stress (e.g., at times of illness or fatigue); they do not necessarily indicate basic pathology. This is also the case during adolescence. Regression serves as a defense, protecting the individual against the intolerable anxiety that genital sexuality arouses. For example, when adults are overwhelmed with anxiety or guilt that cannot be mastered in the face of heterosexual genital sexuality, they may fall back to infantile sexuality—repressing genital sexuality with some prephallic form, and thus developing a perversion.

In ego regression, the mind reverts to modes of functioning typical of an earlier period. Such reacquisition of old patterns is a typical accompaniment of libidinal regression and occurs in response to a variety of needs arising from internal and external pressures. The many causes of ego regression include unpleasurable feelings, such as anxiety or guilt; mental pathology, as seen in neurotic and psychotic processes; and bodily pathology, especially that of the central nervous system and/or that resulting from the disorganization of functioning caused by illness, high fever, or substance abuse. The concept of regression is intimately related to the hypothesis that in the course of attaining adulthood, an individual passes through a series of maturational phases, each with a phase-appropriate mental organization. The makeup of each such organization is inferred from the way instinctual drives discharge, ego functions operate, and conscience and ideals guide behaviors. Under stress or trouble with successful management of the age-appropriate maturational stage, there is a disruption of mental functioning and regression occurs. For instance, a college senior who is achieving well in school fears graduation and career choices, and regresses to the earlier dysfunctional patterns and academic poor performance of early adolescence (which at that time necessitated seeking treatment). Despite enormous therapeutic and academic gains from therapy, the demands of adult life after college pose a threat sufficient to cause substantial regression.

In the course of an assessment, some important questions center on determining whether the current level of functioning is the highest reached, or whether a higher level of adaptation has been abandoned regressively for an earlier one. Nagera (1964) states that "fixation points indicate a certain degree of arrest in drive development. In regressive phenomena, on the other hand, the drives have at one point or another reached a higher level of development but were, as a result of conflicts at these higher levels, forced back to earlier developmental points" (p. 224). The higher the level of development originally attained, the better the prognosis. Nagera suggests that fixations and regressions can be assessed by observing children's behavior, games, play, attitudes, interests, fantasies, and symptoms. In addition, background material presented by parents serves to clarify, confirm, or correct these observations. When evaluating adolescents and adults, clinicians commonly do an ego and superego assessment, and attempt to evaluate age-appropriate, regressed, or faulty functioning (as evident in management of drive expression, frustration tolerance, reality testing, object relations, school and work demands, values and ideals, etc.).

More recent psychoanalytic models, such as self psychology, offer a different explanation of regression. Kohut and his colleagues rejected the conflict model of drive theory and ego psychology, and specifically rejected the notion of instinctual drives as primary motivating forces. "To be able to indicate one's sexual needs, convey one's views and wishes assertively, or to become angry or even aggressive in the face of significant frustration, interference or rejection are expressions of an intact, robust self. That is, experience and expression of healthy instincts are instrumental in the rigorous pursuit of the aims and goals of the self" (Bacal, 1990, p. 235). It was Kohut's view that parents' responses, not the ego or the drives (i.e., libidinal and aggressive drives), determine whether there are deficits in the self of the developing child. "Empathic failure on the part of selfobjects results in deficits; the energy of the drive remains outside of the forming self, giving rise to [regression], driven thoughts or behaviors" (Elson, 1986, p. 37). No single event or trauma creates disorders of the self; rather, the ongoing emotional tone in a family, as well as the impact of parents' specific personalities on the child's subjective experience, produces the self-disorders classified by Kohut and Wolf (1978) as "primary" and "secondary" disorders.

Secondary disorders are reactive disorders that arise in response to the vicissitudes of life and cause depression, grief, or (more commonly) a sense of emptiness, rage, and futility. In some cases, an experience of regression, fragmentation, and depletion occurs in response to a loss, illness, career disappointment, or separation. Commonly, following the trauma and injury to the individual's self-esteem, the individual regains equilibrium with the passage of time, the support of significant selfobjects, and/or significant immersion in work or satisfying activities. Primary disorders of the self include psychoses, borderline states, narcissistic personality, and character disorders, all of which are more prone to repeated regression and fragmentation. Tolpin (1980) noted that impulsivity, drug use, self-injurious behaviors, and shifting object ties represent desperate attempts to cover numerous deficits in self-esteem regulation and in affect/mood management.

There is no reconciling these contrasting paradigms, but it is suggested that each provides useful perspectives in understanding fixation, regression, and defenses. Kohut's emphasis on nature versus nurture, and his focusing on the actual mother and her successes and failures in empathic parenting, are central to his consideration of *reactive* responses of rage, regression, and fragmentation as evidence of self-disorders. The "clinical application of Kohut's theory requires that the therapist move from a classic, silent or interpretive observer role to provide a warmer, more soothing analytic climate" (Mishne, 1993, p. 387). Critical of the detached, neutral observer who offers interpretations from an "experience-distant" position, Kohut (1959, 1982, 1984) emphasized that the clinician should engage in "experience-near" empathy; that is, through the use of vicarious introspection, the clinician should concentrate on trying to understand the patient's subjective perspective, rather than on providing his or her view of external, objective reality.

DEFENSES

Defenses are manifested in a myriad of forms, via habitual modes of relating, acting out, and nonverbal expression. "Defense" is a general term used to describe a struggle of the ego to protect itself against danger. Classic theory states that the danger arises because of the threat of eruption into consciousness of a repressed wish that has become associated with painful feelings of anxiety or guilt—feelings that impel the ego to ward off the wish or drive. Defenses or defense mechanisms occur and operate unconsciously, so that the individual is unaware of what is taking place. Not infrequently, when excessive defenses are called into action, there is a deletion or distortion of defense mechanisms. The examination of defense organization involves assessing whether a defense is employed specifically against individual drives, or more generally against drive activity and instinctual phases. In addition, one must consider whether the defenses are age-adequate, too primitive, or too precocious; and whether they deal effectively with anxiety and depression, or result in disequilibrium, lability, mobility, or deadlock within the structure (A. Freud, 1946, 1951, 1971; Eissler, Freud, Kris, & Solnit, 1977).

The defenses of patients who lack inner structure are due to ego deficits rather than fear and guilt. For example, a borderline patient's impulsive acting out is commonly due to impaired ego functioning (e.g., poor frustration tolerance, poor drive modulation, and a lack of internalized self-soothing mechanisms). The primitive defense of "splitting" mirrors the borderline patient's defective object relations and lack of object constancy (Blanck & Blanck, 1979b). Thus objects are perceived as all-good, all-bad, or ever-changing in terms of cathexis. The patient lacks tolerance for ambivalence, and attachment does not remain constant in the face of frustration. The patient cannot remain irrevocably attached, regardless of gratification.

An absence of defenses is a serious danger sign. If a defense against anxiety is lacking or completely unsuccessful, the patient suffers panic attacks or full-blown anxiety attacks, both of which are harmful for the overwhelmed ego. The occurrence of these states is indicative of a failure to acquire the important ability to reduce anxiety to structurally useful "signal anxiety" (i.e., the smaller amount necessary to stimulate appropriate defensive response).

Many specific types of defenses have been identified. Among these, in addition to "splitting," are the following:

- "Denial" is a primitive defense mechanism whereby the ego avoids becoming aware of some painful reality. The disagreeable or unwelcome fact is thereby erased.
- "Projection" is another primitive defense, in which unwelcome thoughts or feelings are attributed outside the self.
- A more advanced defense is "displacement," the transfer of hostile feelings from one person to another (e.g., from a family member to a friend, an authority figure, or a therapist).
- "Reaction formation" is the replacement in conscious awareness of a painful idea or feeling by its opposite (e.g., a child's hatred and resentment of a new sibling is repressed, and the child shows the new sibling extreme solicitude and concern).
- "Isolation of affect" may be manifested in compartmentalized thinking (e.g., emotional events are recalled minus the appropriate accompanying affect).
- "Identification with the aggressor" is evidenced by an individual's emulating the feared and aggressive father, in peer and sibling relationships.
- "Reversal of affect" may be exemplified by the relating of a sad event in a pleased and happy manner.
- "Sublimation" is a high-level defense involving the neutraliza-

tion of and transformation of drives, ego energies, and sense of self into activities that promote cohesion and creativity. Examples include immersion in academics, work, sports, artistic or musical efforts, or other activities that are conflict-free.

• "Intellectualization" and "rationalization" are used to attempt to provide emotional distance from overwhelming affects, moods, stimuli, and feelings.

• "Withdrawal" into solitude is often an attempt to ward off painful acknowledgment of personal or familial problems and inadequacies.

• "Acting out" is a displacement of behavioral response from one situation to another. It is the partial discharge of drive tension that is achieved by responding to the present situation as if it were the situation that originally gave rise to the drive demand. It is more than a single thought or expression; it is real action, and can constitute character structure if it is a chronic or habitual pattern of reaction (e.g., explosiveness, hysterics, or impotence at the slightest correction or criticism; see below).

• "Undoing" is an expiatory act that alters another act. Specifically, it is the opposite of something against which the ego must defend itself (e.g., a father wishes to be a better disciplinarian, but then overindulges his child out of unacceptable guilt or feeling of rage at the child).

"Character defense" is a type of defense that defines an individual's total personality. It represents a specific way of being and is an expression of the total past. The four main types of character defense are (1) "hysterical," (2) "compulsive," (3) "phallic–narcissistic," and (4) "masochistic." The following descriptions of these four types are based on Campbell (1981, p. 150):

1. The hysterical or histrionic personality displays vanity and egocentric, attention-seeking antics. Dramatic self-presentation is commonly evident, as are overtalkativeness, excitability, and demanding and manipulative patterns.

2. The compulsive character can have a fanatic concern for orderliness, and a tendency to collect and hoard things. Thinking can be ruminative and obsessive. This type of character armor is generally a defense against sadistic and aggressive impulses.

3. The phallic–narcissistic character can appear self-confident and arrogant; behavior is generally reserved and cold or scornfully aggressive. Phallic–narcissistic attitudes in men are attributed to the need to defend against passive feminine tendencies and represent an unconscious rage against the opposite sex. The narcissistic character also involves chronic tendencies to be self-damaging and self-depreciating.

4. The masochistic character is a defense against punishment. Anxiety is avoided by overgiving and by excessive toleration of abuse, out of a desire to be loved.

Here again, self psychology posits a different basis for defensive activity, which is not viewed as a protective armor against dangerous drives and wishes. Defenses are viewed as attempts to protect the self from significant psychological injury, such as a repetition of traumatic assaults on self-esteem that occurred in childhood. Thus Kohut preferred to consider defensiveness in treatment as a rekindled fear, not as a indication of "resistance" to treatment. There is a dread of "being re-traumatized by one's bad objects as represented by the [therapist and the treatment]" (Bacal, 1990, p. 221), as had occurred in early life at the hands of nonempathic, unattuned parents. Defenses are seen as arising out of anxious anticipation or actual experience with therapeutic ruptures in the course of treatment. Defenses are thus viewed as existing in the relational context of past and present object relations, rather than as lodged in the individual, who is responding to fears about dangerous wishes and forbidden drive expression. "Protracted resistance (and defensiveness) to the analytic work, or negative therapeutic reaction is regarded as being due to the patient's experience of the analyst's persistent empathic lag or out-of-tuneness with the patient's primary self-disorders and self-object needs" (Bacal, 1979; see also Brandchaft, 1983).

CASE OF MIKE: EXAMPLE OF FIXATION, REGRESSION, AND DEFENSES IN WORK WITH AN AFRICAN AMERICAN LATENCY-AGE CHILD

Referral

When Mike was 10½ years old, the social worker at his school referred him to a child psychiatry clinic for evaluation. Mike was described as a bright child who read far above grade level, but regressed and acted younger than his age, and stubbornly refused to produce in school. He refused to participate in class discussions or to interact with peers, and his teachers often felt at their wits' end with him. The school had just failed him on the basis of his refusal to work. In previous years he had been passed not because of his performance, but on the basis of his obvious intellect. The parents projected Mike's problems onto the school and various teachers; they had considered sending him to a private school, but after making inquiries, they determined that the cost of private education was prohibitive. Though they acknowledged problems at home with Mike, their conscious perception of the situation was that their son was of superior intellect, was bored in class, and had been mishandled by his teachers. The father was also concerned about Mike's manliness, due to his "dumb," unhearing affect and his refusal to defend himself with peers.

History of Presenting Complaints

When Mike entered kindergarten at age 5, he was "disappointed" at not being taught to read "big books." He already demonstrated more than basic reading skills. The parents stated that he complained about coloring projects and the curriculum or lack thereof, but did well socially. In the first grade, his teacher had to leave suddenly before the end of the spring semester, and Mike stopped doing any work. In the second grade, he obtained good marks, but only because he had been forced to work; on several occasions he came home with bruised buttocks and descriptions of paddlings. His teachers complained that getting him to work was "like pulling teeth." The parents were extremely upset about the spankings and contacted the teachers. However, they subsequently skirted the issue about the punitive handling of Mike, as they were preoccupied with the sudden death of the maternal grandmother from a stroke.

Mike changed schools in the third grade and was placed in a combination second- and third-grade class. He complained of having to repeat work he had had the year before. Despite his resistance and refusal to comply with any assignments, he passed. The spring before his referral, when Mike was in the fourth grade, the school failed him on the basis of his refusal to work. The mother said that the school faculty members felt very frustrated with Mike and couldn't decide whether he should repeat the fourth grade or be skipped to the sixth grade. Over the summer, the parents forced Mike to participate in summer school, hoping he could avoid repeating the fourth grade. Mike was still in summer school when the referral for evaluation was made.

Mike was an attractive, well-built, very light-skinned black boy with a slow, cautious smile. He presented like a little adult; ignoring all toys, he talked nonstop, finding it difficult to end each interview. Mike's own account of school conformed with the description given by the referring school social worker and his parents. He was bored in school and had not made any warm attachments to teachers or peers. He was openly fearful of peers, got bullied, and was unable to fight back and defend himself. He was aware of his father's anger at his cowardice, which made him feel ashamed. He could not even defend himself against one of his high-spirited younger sisters. He was closest to his mother and planned to study piano (her profession was teaching the piano). He had few good friends; in fact, he referred to only two nonthreatening peers in the neighborhood. One was a boy much younger than Mike, and the other was a crippled child with whom he spent much time. He seemed to experience little pleasure or mastery in play or in school. Summer school was seen as better than regular school because of a variety of interesting trips. However, Mike seemed to feel no consistent, internalized pleasure or confident sense of self in any sphere of life. Fear of his parents' tempers, as well as of his own temper, was a major theme. Mike conveyed a lonely, angry, and fearful self-concept: that of a "sissy" (his word) who strongly repressed his anger and self-assertion, profoundly feared his father, and identified with his mother (whom he favored).

Family Background

Mike's father was an attractive, vital, humorous, warm black man. He had less formal education than his wife, having spent only a year or so at a community college. He worked as a traffic manager in a factory and as a part-time TV repairman, to try to make ends meet. He worked long hours, getting home late four nights a week. He was rarely home except on weekends, when he slept, watched sports on TV, or ran some errands. He and his wife made a rather incongruous couple. She was very small, light-skinned, tense, intellectual, and formal, while he was darker-complexioned, earthy, open, and relaxed. The parents owned their own home but struggled to manage financially, with the mother giving piano lessons at home. The mother said there was no time or money for socializing with friends. The family appeared to be socially isolated.

The parents had been married 11 years earlier, when the mother was 20 and the father was 30. He had been married before, when he was 17. That first marriage had lasted 11 years and produced five children; the oldest was now 23 and the youngest was 16. The father said that his first wife, always "something of a drinker," began to frequent taverns all night after their fifth child was born; she would take money from her wealthy father and leave her husband home with the laundry and the care of the five children. She had her father buy them a lavish home and pay for maids, while she "caroused, had affairs, and smashed up cars with her drunken driving." Her sisters raised the children after the divorce, although the father said he was actively involved in the children's lives, paying child support and seeing them several times a week. He stated that four out of the five had turned out well; only the youngest had problems. He was described as unreachable, stubborn, and rebellious. The father said that he had finally terminated this hellish first marriage out of fear that he would go out of control and beat his wife. He said he had always struggled to control himself. When he was 13, he had broken a boy's jaw in a furious fight. He maintained relationships with his in-laws from the first marriage, and in fact was employed by his ex-father-in-law.

The father met his second wife (Mike's mother) at work. He was drawn to her because she seemed to be the exact opposite of his first wife. He said he was happy that she was a homemaker and conscientious about their children, although "she's a temperamental musician and not always the easiest to get along with." The parents seemed to have preserved their marriage through using substantial repression and denial. Finances were a chronic problem, and the mother was very critical about her husband's expenditures and over-spending on cars, clothes, a boat, and toys for the children. She kept her income separate, using it for household and personal items.

Developmental History and Further Family History

Mike, who was conceived immediately after the marriage, was not planned but was "accepted," despite both parents' concerns about finances and the father's obligations to support the children of his first marriage. The mother continued working as a bookkeeper through a comfortable pregnancy. Delivery was full-term with a normal labor. The mother nursed Mike for 5 to 6 months, and he was described as a quiet, easy baby who ate and slept well and was very responsive. He never used a pacifier or sucked his thumb. He was weaned from the bottle at 1 year, though his grandmother gave the bottle back at 14 months when his first sister (also unplanned) was born. Mike was described as being curious but not jealous of the new baby and as playing gently with her. The mother had gone back to work when Mike was 6 months old, leaving him in the care of her mother. She returned to work 3 months after the birth of the second child; Mike was then 17 months old.

The mother stated that her employment had been necessary, given the father's child support obligations; she felt positive about her mother's care of her children, since her mother was young and lively, and had young children of her own (Mike's mother was the oldest of six). Once two more girls were born, the mother curtailed her outside employment. She described finding teaching piano at home to be a mixed blessing. She resented not getting out at all, and yet she also liked being able to supervise her children better, as well as not having to commute to work or spend money on lunch, carfare, and sitters. The mother enjoyed making music more than she enjoyed teaching it. She shared her enjoyment and frustration with music. She claimed to have been a child prodigy who began piano lessons at age 3, at which time she also learned to read. She won a music scholarship to college, but had to give it up and go to work after 1 year. She never returned to college and gave her earnings to her parents for a down payment on a home.

Despite her closeness with her mother, the mother's life in her family of origin was a painful one, which affected her handling of her own children. As the oldest of six children, she had little privacy and was never allowed to express any aggression. She was smacked by her mother for any sign of anger (e.g., slamming a door). She tearfully acknowledged to me that her current even temper and blandness in public were "a show and a cover-up." In private when she was upset, she erupted—throwing dishes, kicking furniture, slamming doors, yelling, and crying. Her parents had fought a great deal over money, and she worried that this was being replicated in her fights with her husband about family finances. The mother said that because she was always precocious intellectually and musically, she had always received a lot of support and money for dancing and piano lessons, which she felt guilty about. Despite her struggles about assertiveness, she was close to her mother, who encouraged her interests and was proud of her abilities. Since her mother's shocking and unexpected death 2 years earlier, she had been concerned about her youngest two (high-school-age) sisters, who refused to live with her and were left almost completely unsupervised as their father pursued a string of women.

The father's traumatic history had also somewhat adversely affected his involvement with his children, especially Mike. His dad had died when he was 4 months old. His mother went on public assistance and later worked as a maid. He was raised jointly by his mother, aunt, and grandmother, whom he described as "black, Southern, superstitious, church-going, ladies." He was made to participate in church activities, such as selling flowers and churning ice cream for church socials and banquets. His aunt had five sons who were like brothers to him. His aunt was separated from her husband, but strict in supervising her sons and him. Being one of the youngest, he got away with a lot, since his aunt was warm and indulgent (she had taught him to read at age 3); however, her indulgence alternated with her explosions. Out of exhaustion, when her patience ran out, she would often severely spank him.

The father had worked from early childhood on, selling ice and coal for his movie and spending money. When he was 9 years old, his mother married a seemingly quiet, church-going man who could only earn a meager living in the steel mills, so his mother had to continue to work as a maid. His stepfather had a son 4 years older, who was described as "mean and selfish." In conflict with his stepbrother and stepfather, he left home at age 13 and lived on his own in a rented room, going to high school, and visiting his mother once a month. When he was about 16 years old, his stepfather died of a stroke, and his mother moved in with cousins; she continued to work as a maid. He saw his mother when he wasn't out socializing and gambling. He said he didn't dare drink for fear of losing his temper, but he made quite a bit of money gambling and playing pool and cards. He did well academically and had plans for college. He had many girlfriends but avoided male friends, stating that boys his age were only interested in drinking, drugs, and drifting, whereas he stayed in his room, studying and listening to opera. In his fourth year of high school, he got a girl pregnant; he quit school to work, finished high school (and briefly attended a community college) at night, and married the girl when they were both 17 years old. The father recounted much of this to me with humor, zest, and pride that he got through it all.

Mike's father and mother related warmly and well throughout the evaluation process. They were relieved that Mike had also connected with me, and did not complain about having appointments twice a week at the clinic. Both parents, with support, responded well to preliminary parent guidance. For his part, Mike continued to evidence no interest in toys in the clinic playroom; rather, he still presented like a little adult, pouring out relevant information about his problems at home and at school. Mike impressed both the clinic's student psychologist and me as a very anxious latency-age child who had adopted a passive–aggressive stance to minimize anxiety conjured up by threatening stimuli and circumstances. Retreat, withdrawal, and passive–aggressive reactions characterized his general behavior. Intellectual and psychological tests showed a boy of very good endowment but low self-esteem; he was crippled by anxiety to such an extent that he evidenced constricted informational input, and had difficulty in planning, anticipating, and interpreting social situations. Despite his intelligence and capacity for abstraction, he failed to perceive and recognize the big picture or total situation. Other tests suggested difficulty in dealing with affect. Though he constantly reminded one of his intellectual capacities, at a deeper level he felt afraid, lonely, and different, and was alienated by marked feelings of inferiority. Part of this poor self-concept was his view of himself as unable to fight or run fast like other boys his age. He expressed ambivalence about all peer interactions; in particular, he voiced shame about being a very light-complexioned African American child in an urban city school serving peers who were darker, and seemingly (in his eyes) more masculine, than he was. He fantasized grandiose achievements with wishes to perform well and to be powerful and successful. The challenges of imminent puberty and sexual identity overwhelmed Mike, who saw the world as hostile and attacking.

Diagnostic Assessment of Mike

A TRADITIONAL PSYCHOANALYTIC PERSPECTIVE

Mike's ego was intact. There were no signs or symptoms of primary defects. Nor were there signs of primary deficiencies in his ego functions. His memory, reality testing, speech, and secondary thought processes reflected intactness. He was an intelligent boy who scored well on achievement tests, but he withheld and would not produce in school. There was secondary interference of his defense symptoms with many of his ego functions. His overall defense organization consisted of repression, fixation, and regression to anal levels; specific defenses included reaction formation, marked withdrawal, and turning of aggression against the self. These defenses seemed to be a response to his totally inadequate Oedipal resolution and lack of masculine identification. Mike's ineffective defenses caused anxiety and ego regression, which interfered with his social and academic adjustment. His learning was not basically impaired, but his refusal to produce in school and at home infuriated the adults in his environment and resulted in emotional and physical abusiveness and a sado-masochistic interpersonal mode of relating. Either Mike had entered the phallic–Oedipal phase and regressed to an anal level, or he was fixated at the anal (stubborn) level of development. His profound anal withholding in school supposedly began after a teacher's sudden departure, experienced as "abandonment." The grandmother's sudden death was probably the actual significant abandonment, since he had been "placed" with her and she was his original primary caregiver. His repeated "loss" of his natural mother occurred via this placement with the grandmother and the rapid succession of siblings, born so close together.

Mike feared his parents' aggressiveness, yet stimulated them to act out aggressively toward him, in a manner characteristic of an anal sado-masochistic pattern. His superego, like his ego, seemed regressed, with little guilt discernible. The parents' explosiveness frightened Mike away from an open expression of anger in a safe environment. His punitive superego was rigid and maladaptive, creating a constant need for punishment. Mike was ambivalently connected to his mother, a warm and intelligent woman involved in his intellectual and cultural development (e.g., with music), but she also frightened him because of her depression and explosive temper. He thwarted her hopes for his academic success and her wish that he mirror her childhood achievements in school; thus he could not maintain a positive inner image of his mother. Instead, he was clinging, controlling, and withholding. Because he appeared regressed to or fixated at the anal phase, he was unable to please or identify with his reproachful, generally absent father, who was angry, disappointed in him, impatient, and often explosive. Mike recoiled not only from his father, but also from all sports and activities valued by the father as exciting masculine games. Mike said that he feared body contact sports, since he indeed feared physical confrontations with peers, many of which he provoked—especially when he downplayed or even demeaned black identity, black curriculum content in school, black musicians, and the like. Mike lauded his Native American ancestors and claimed to be Native American, not African American. Although there was one Native American great-grandparent, his parents' and his primary lineage appeared to be African American. This selected self-identification was yet another avenue Mike unconsciously used, seemingly to distance himself from his dad, whom he so feared prior to treatment (when he was spanked constantly).

Mike's entry into latency was greatly compromised by the above-noted fixations and regression. He evidenced external conflict between the aggressive drive and the object world, and internal conflicts between his ego and superego, both arousing fear of the object world. Mike had not progressed very far from the dependent position or toward age-appropriate object relationships. In the mornings, he had to be prodded to get up, get dressed, and get in motion. He dawdled and showed little independence. He learned seemingly by osmosis, withholding any compliance with routine schoolwork. Adults were infuriated by this bright boy's refusal to participate. He had no hobbies or evident interests or pleasures. His conflicts with his environment were profound. Little would be accomplished by simple environmental manipulation (e.g., a school change), since Mike would undoubtedly manifest the same problems in any new school setting, even a benign one. Clearly he needed treatment, which would need to include work with his parents to modify their handling of their son. Long-term fairly extensive psychotherapy was indicated, based on the long-standing nature of Mike's withholdingness. It was likely that he might become stubborn, withholding, and testing, provoking any therapist. It might well take him time to establish a trusting relationship of depth, given the extent of his stressful connection to his parents. He could be so infuriating that teachers, like his parents, confessed to spanking him; even the clinic's student psychologist ruefully acknowledged yelling at and scolding him during the assessment process. He was diagnosed as having a character disorder of the passive–aggressive type, with depressive and narcissistic features.

A SELF-PSYCHOLOGICAL PERSPECTIVE

Although I will not attempt to integrate the more traditional psychoanalytic findings summarized above with self psychology, what follows is a discussion of the assessment of Mike and his parents from a self-psychological perspective. I concur with Ornstein's (1983) objections to efforts to integrate self psychology into the more traditional perspectives: "One either views the developmental line of narcissism as separate, with all of the clinical and theoretical consequences of such a view, or one chooses not to view it as separate with all its consequences" (p. 383). Despite the lack of (possible) integration, I believe that varied models offer different and useful clinical data.

At the time of the referral and beginning of treatment, Mike and his parents each could be viewed as having a primary disturbance of the self. An individual with a disorder of the self exists in states of varying degrees of coherence, from cohesion to fragmentation; in states of varying degrees of functional harmony, from order to chaos; and in states of varying degrees of vitality, from vigor to enfeeblement. Significant failure to achieve cohesion, vigor, or harmony, or a significant loss of these qualities after they have been tentatively established, may be said to constitute a state of self-disorder (Kohut & Wolf, 1978). Mike and his parents each presented as seriously damaged, chaotic, and explosive, and the parents together could best be described as selfobjects to Mike and each other in considerable disarray. Each family member commonly exhibited cycles of attacks of "scathing narcissistic rage, i.e., selfishly demanding rage attacks on one another, with seeming oblivion to the rights and feelings of those toward whom their demands are directed" (Kohut & Wolf, 1978, p. 193). Clearly underlying each family member's rage was a pervasive sense of enfeeblement, hopelessness, and helplessness.

Mike's structural deficits caused "faulty self-esteem, a missing sense of direction, inadequately formed ideals, fragmentation anxiety and depression" (Tolpin, 1978, p. 181). The lack of structure occurred because Mike's parents could not and did not provide optimal frustration; the parental selfobjects were not in tune with his needs and wishes, and impervious to his needs for "affirmation, confirmation and guidance" (Elson, 1986, p. 91).

Additional to the above-noted characteristics are the following suggested by Beren (1998) when one is considering narcissistic pathology in childhood. The first of these is overvaluation of the self, with the corresponding need for constant admiration, attention, and/or self-aggrandizement, or a need to devalue others. Grandiosity may be expressed by a sense of specialness and/or entitlement, or in other ways in which the child sees him- or herself as hero. Second, undervaluation of the self is frequently manifested in expressions of feeling emotionally upset, easily injured, inferior, ashamed, and/or worthless. Third, an exaggerated need for the selfobject is often evidenced by a child's requiring a mirroring, exclusively dyadic relationship in order to maintain an ideal state of self. In addition, though desperately needy for others' attention, children with self-disorders generally lack self-awareness and empathy for themselves and for the needs and feelings of others. Narcissistic children also lack the flexibility for easy play and for the rough-and-tumble of peer relationships. Finally, their precocious ego development and (often) high intelligence cause great unevenness in development; consequently, parents, teachers, and peers often suffer confusion and endless frustration in their expectations of and interactions with such children (Beren, 1998).

Treatment

Mike's parents were responsive to parent guidance. Relieved that they were not alone in their struggles with their son, they were able to alter their handling of him quickly and dramatically. They were helped to distance themselves in order to avoid aggressive outbursts (i.e., fierce scoldings and physical discipline). They learned to walk away and not engage in power struggles; for example, by shutting Mike's door and tolerating his messy room, they could curtail yelling, screaming, and spanking him. They were helped to talk out, rather than act out, their upset and anger.

Mike was seen twice a week and sometimes three times a week over a 4 year period. The parents were amazed and relieved that getting him out the door for early-morning therapy sessions was not a problem, since Mike's motivation for help stimulated him not to dawdle and drag his feet (as he did in all other areas of his life) in leaving the home. Mike brought material into treatment in various ways. He was very verbal and articulate; he also spent much time drawing, and ultimately sharing, fantasies and associations (see below). Initially, he presented an excessive amount of verbal content, much of which was a series of rationalizations, intellectualizations, and projections. He resisted any comment, reflection, or interpretation about his regressed state; instead, he kept up his endless barrage, seemingly needing to ensure control and to defend against his fear of expressing aggression, as well as to keep me as the therapist at a safe distance. I responded to his need for admiration, and ceased making observations and/or interpretations he seemingly only could reject or ignore. He clearly was struggling with his wish for and fear of closeness, his sibling rivalry, and his fear of failure. Mike needed pacification and responded positively to my efforts to soothe, empathize, and employ vicarious introspection. "Perceiving the [patient's] state of mind, his immediate and general way of experiencing himself and others, his range of feelings and thoughts, is of course the critical task of treatment, but to do so requires the greatest discipline" (Lichtenberg, 1983, pp. 164–165). In working with Mike, it was clear that he hungered for more active listening, mirroring, soothing, undivided attention. These were not possible in his home, given the abundance of children—not only his more needy three younger siblings, but his demanding adolescent and young adult half-siblings from his father's first marriage.

During the first year of therapy, Mike acknowledged his wish to be my best and favorite child. He acted out his feelings of sibling rivalry in his competition with a youngster I saw the hour before his appointment. He would joke and laugh as he related checking out whether "that little noisy girl is also seeing you today." He looked for her, or for telltale signs (e.g., scraps of colored paper) that had been overlooked in "cleanup" before his arrival. He feared his angry feelings toward this girl, as well as toward his actual siblings at home. His alarm about his own angry impulses was externalized into elaborate fears of tornadoes, floods, fires, storms, and planes or lightning crashing into the clinic. He drew endless, obsessively detailed, exact renderings of airplanes, trains, racing cars, ships, and monsters. His running dialogue accompanying his drawings was a gradual sharing of omnipotent, megalomaniac fantasies related to his drawings of the day, or sometimes to a GI Joe doll he often brought into treatment sessions. Over time Mike's drawings became more and more ordered and skillfully drawn, and gradually more reflective of age-appropriate interests. Beautifully drawn guitars and references to musical groups replaced his prior obsession with monsters, mystery planes, ships, and so on.

Mike made significant gains after 2 years of therapy. His schoolwork improved rapidly, and his academic achievement consistently reached a superior level. Mike also moved from a state of social and familial isolation, passivity, and femininity to a more active, age-appropriate, somewhat more comfortable masculine self-presentation. He was less provocative both at home and at school, and slowly began to participate in swimming classes and on a Little League baseball team.

When his and my different racial identities were discussed, to explore whether this fed into his disavowal of his African American identity and preference to be viewed as Native American, Mike was amused. He pointed out to me that his mother and I shared the same skin tone, and that in the summer when I tanned, I appeared to be more African American than his mother. Mike was able to talk at length about the reality of his being ostracized and teased by peers because of his light skin tone. Referring to his similarly light-skinned siblings and mother, Mike reflected the reality that "skin color can (and does) evoke very powerful and painful feelings among African-Americans that strike at the core of their identity and self-esteem" (Williams, 1996, p. 211). This physical characteristic of light skin color estranged Mike from his darker-complexioned peers, father, and half-siblings, and placed him with the females (his mother and younger sisters), the other light-skinned members of the family. Thus Mike evidenced an unconscious feminine identity and a low level of racial identity development (Atkinson, Morten, & Sue, 1998), characterized by self-depreciating attitudes and beliefs.

Mike's features of puberty and early adolescence were minimal; like many boys his age, he lagged in physical development, which caused him some self-consciousness. Despite some improved contact with peers after the first 2 years of therapy, in his search for a new love object he ignored his peers and fastened onto me, preferring my company to that of all others. The transference appeared to have a selfobject basis, initially for merger-mirroring, and later for idealization. He articulated a wish for daily sessions, and ultimately, with some degree of resentful resignation, accepted an increase from twice-weekly to thrice-weekly appointments. My countertransference reactions were a complicated mix of powerful positive maternal feelings and routine awe and amazement, in response to Mike's demonstration of his remarkable intellectual and creative talents. On other occasions, empathy and vicarious introspection caused me to feel lonely and sad, hopeless and helpless, as I struggled with my own sense of frustration that this gifted and talented child was so estranged and so alone outside the office. Only in my office was he clearly at his best in terms of appropriate behavior, growing positive attachment, and comfort level; here he was able to be creative, intellectually curious, and psychologically minded. Wishing that I could see him four or five times a week—as he wanted, and as I believe would have been ideal—caused me to feel frustrated. I knew such frequency could not be managed by Mike's parents. As it was, bringing him two to three times a week was often all but overwhelming, given the reality needs of their other children and the father's work demands.

In the period where Mike was seen three times a week, he made more gains and seemed able to move forward at a faster pace. Mike demonstrated increased capacities for self-observation and intro- spection. He was able to verbalize feelings and fantasies more freely. He could articulate his belief that my reflections and explanations had helped him figure things out—

"like my imagination baby games and heroes, full of monsters, racing cars, stars, and pilots. I used to like to lose myself in my daydreams, thinking about those make-believe people, because I'm the opposite and want to feel good and forget that I'm the shortest in my class, not popular, not a big shot, not a good ath- lete, and too frightened to fight and defend myself. Now I'm an excellent student, and it's the only thing in my control. I guess I'm just all brains and no brawn."

In his early adolescent identification with me, Mike spoke of be- coming a therapist and often read about psychological matters, con- sulting encyclopedias and library books. With a twinkle in his eye, Mike often spoke of reading a book about Freud, in which there was a story about a grown man afraid of the dark because he had been locked in a closet as a child when punished. The man was also afraid of dogs, and the book, according to Mike, stated that the fear of dogs was really a substitute for or displacement from his fear of his par- ents. Mike then would ponder the meaning of his own fears—of bugs, a ball coming at him in a game, tackles or blows in contact team sports, or other unexpected events—and their significance as displacements from his intense earlier fears of his dad, who used to spank him severely.

With the overall gains that Mike was making, he clearly showed that he had moved from the regressed position where he had been fixated. He resumed a progressive line of development and slowly but surely dealt with his long-standing anger, sibling rivalry, and feelings of abandonment caused by his care's having been turned over to his grandmother and the births of three younger siblings in rapid succession. Most significant was his ability to come to terms with the original trauma (the death of his grandmother) that had led to his developmental arrest and fixations.

Blos (1962) observed the uneven rite of passage through the adolescent period, noting the continual progressions, regressions, and digressions. "The adolescent may rush through these various phases or he may elaborate on any one of them in endless variations but he cannot altogether sidestep the essential psychic transformations of the various phases" (pp. 52–53). Despite Mike's significant gains in therapy, becoming a teenager produced considerable stress and regression once he entered "adolescence proper" (i.e., middle adolescence, ages 14–17).

> The phase of adolescence proper has two dominant themes: the revival of the Oedipal complex and the disengagement from primary love objects. This process constitutes a sequence of object-relinquishment and object finding, both of which promote the establishment of the adult drive organization. One may describe this phase of adolescence in terms of two broad affective stages; "mourning and being in love." The adolescent incurs a real loss in the renunciation of his Oedipal parents and he experiences the inner emptiness, grief, and sadness which [are] part of all mourning. (Blos, 1962, p. 100)

The disengagement from parents and the process of mourning noted by Blos commonly cause regression to earlier arrests or fixation points during adolescence. Sometimes, "out of their own needs, parents seek to halt development. . . . In other instances, fearing separation and the task of self-definition, adolescents may linger in a merger which does not permit that quickening opportunity for trusting and expanding their perceptions, for initiating a unique program of action which is the necessary task of these years" (Elson, 1984, p. 311).

As Mike entered middle adolescence, there was a short-lived regressive decline in his superior academic achievements. In particular, his argumentativeness with teachers resurfaced. Mike would engage his teachers in power struggles over assignments and the curriculum; he would try to trip them up on obscure scientific data;

and/or he would depreciate black studies content (assignments related to Martin Luther King, the history of slavery, the NAACP, Angela Davis, etc.). He would provocatively refuse to do homework and simple assignments. Mike was aware of his conflictual feelings regarding his own racial identity, which were manifested in both fantasies about his actual Native American ancestor, and his wish to be European or Native American rather than African American. Mike reverted to obsessive drawings and ruminations, and was generally ambivalent about active–passive conflicts and masculine–feminine issues. He also demonstrated the heightened self-consciousness of adolescence, in his preoccupation with his short stature and his new interest in guitar playing. He drew endless intricate pictures of guitars, session after session; as of old, he entertained some childlike grandiose fantasies about overnight megasuccess as a musician (an activity he actually devoted little time to). He acknowledged being seduced by the hype and monied success of rock stars.

Mike was also preoccupied with his independent intellectual pursuits and his astoundingly high scores on academic achievement tests, especially in math and science. Though not compliant with all academic expectations and assignments, he soon regained his excellent level of academic success, and was chosen to give a series of science "lectures" or reports. His high scores on achievement tests enabled him to change schools and be admitted to a most competitive and rigorous public school that offered advanced placements in science and math.

DISCUSSION OF ETHNIC/CULTURAL/RACIAL ISSUES IN THE TREATMENT OF MIKE AND HIS PARENTS

From the onset, work with Mike and his parents demonstrated the "intertwining of social issues and internal conflicts that are frequently part of the Black middle-class experience" (Thompson, 1996, p. 188). Mike's father had grown up poor and fatherless in a Southern black community. The strength of the women in the extended family was noteworthy, as demonstrated by the loyalty and commitment of the father's mother, aunt, and grandmother. The father and his aunt's five sons were cared for by these three dedicated, strong women, faced with six boys to raise in a financially deprived fatherless milieu. This sort of matriarchial home is not uncommon in the lives of African American clients.

Mike's father had worked from an early age with no respite, despite his mother's remarriage to a low-wage-earning millhand when he was 9 years old. In conflict with his stepfather as an adolescent, he moved out of his home and indulged in the unsupervised adult activities of cards, gambling, pool playing, and premature sexual experiences, the last of which resulted in his impregnating a girl. They married when both were 17 years old, and proceeded to have more unplanned children together. There was no consideration of abortion or surrender of a baby for adoption by these black teenage parents.

Mike's mother, the oldest of six children, came from an essentially lower-middle-class working family where skin color was part of the attribution of middle-class status. The mother experienced herself as favored by her mother because of her skin color, intellectual facility, and musical talents. Despite her favorite status, she was roughly disciplined by her overwrought mother, who struggled to manage six children amidst her strife-ridden marriage and precarious financial situation. Mike' mother's musical talents secured her a college scholarship, but she dropped out of school to work, and helped her parents with her earnings and with the care of her younger siblings. Unconsciously, in her own marriage she appeared to be replicating her mother's marriage; like her mother, she had a rapid succession of unplanned children, as well as arguments with her husband regarding expenditures and how monies were designated. She struggled with her temper, as did her husband, especially in their parenting struggles with Mike.

What appeared striking was the degree of relief in Mike's parents' reaction to their son's therapy with me, as well as the rapport and trust that were quickly established between me and the parents. Griffin (1977) notes that a major theme of psychotherapy where the therapist is white and the patient is black is trust. This establishment of trust appeared to be based on the ease we all experienced from the onset in talking together—be it about Mike, their travails in parenting him, their own lives, their marriage, or music (i.e., the mother's musical education and interests, and the father's knowledge and love of opera). Although I am not a professional musician, I happened to share their appreciation of music, and my familiarity with their source of pleasure and solace was apparent. More important, I believe, was the parents' sensing my grasp of their black experience and the extent and impact of their lifelong financial stress (i.e., the father's fatherless childhood of poverty, and the mother's lower-middle-class, "barely making ends meet" existence). Langman (1999) states that "viewing their own immigrant experience as the norm, Jews often expect Blacks to move up the economic ladder the same way earlier generations of Jews moved up. This expectation is based on another misunderstanding, the lack of appreciation of the pervasiveness of racism in America." Julius Lester (1994), an African American convert to Judiasm, has stated: "To cite the immigrant experience as the paradigm is to ignore the legacy of slavery. [It] is also to be blind to the seeming intractability of color prejudice in American society" (pp. 170–171). I believed (and continue to believe) that the parents recognized my lack of expectation of such easy upward mobility, and that they felt my understanding of the economic and psychological hardships of their present life and their childhood experiences.

I believe that Mike's parents and I were able to form a working alliance because I was able to communicate genuine concern for Mike's welfare from the onset, rather than merely viewing him as a disruptive nuisance (as his teachers did). The emphasis throughout was on their own and their son's inner feelings, pain, and confusion. Thus the parents did not experience stigma, concerns about confidentiality, or overwhelming parental guilt. From the onset, we all shared the same psychological conception of the problem. Moreover, the parents did not feel blamed for their physical discipline; rather, they were recognized as anxious, frantic, and bewildered by their son, and by the problems he posed at home and at school. During the thorough and lengthy assessment and history-taking process, I was able to provide preliminary advice and recommendations regarding methods of discipline, age-appropriate behavior, and so on. "Direct advice to parents is seldom effective, unless the parents' attitude towards the child is empathic and this understanding is sufficient to enable them to interact meaningfully with the child" (Sours, 1978, p. 624). I viewed the parents as empathic and motivated, and was not disappointed in this view: Their cooperation over a 4-year period in getting Mike to early-morning appointments, whatever the weather or demands at home, was remarkable. I believe that a solid working alliance is the key to successful engagement and treatment of children and adolescents. Obviously, a successful alliance is devoid of what Hacker (1994) identifies as "benevolent condescension" in cross-racial treatment (e.g., Jews' helping blacks not as equals, but as superiors reaching down to assist the helpless or the needy). This attitude assumes a certain level of inferiority on the part of blacks. It is a form of racism. My respect for Mike's parents' unwavering commitment to secure help for their son was matched, I believe, by their respect for me and our partnership in the work we shared, and by their relief at the gains we all were able to make.

When Mike entered therapy, he appeared to be at a low level of racial identity development, as noted earlier. He evidenced "unequivocal preference for dominant cultural values over [his] own" (Sue & Sue, 1999, p. 129). He conformed to the findings of Clark and Clark (1947), who noted that racism may contribute to a sense of confused self-identity among black children. They found that some black children preferred white dolls, and indeed Mike preferred playing with a white doll (his GI Joe doll) over black ones. He also preferred the music of white musicians over the music of blacks. He scorned black studies content in school and dominant black peer values; this infuriated his peers, who teased and tormented him, and his black teachers, who felt driven to spank him. He attempted to dress like a white youth or a Native American, shunning the hairstyle, clothing, and other aspects of appearance typical of black youths his age. He originally viewed his blackness as a handicap, and attempted to define himself as nonblack, conveying a belief system in which nonblack standards were viewed as superior. He resented his hair texture and other African American features, and preferred his light skin color. It was abundantly clear that for Mike, skin color served "various aspects of psychic organization" (Thompson, 1996, p. 126). Because his father was dark-complexioned and his mother was very light-skinned, Mike's light skin color also posed gender identity issues for him: It was viewed as contributing to his non-athletic, sports-avoidant, feminine stance, which disappointed and enraged his father and alarmed his mother.

According to Boyd-Franklin (1991), the issue of skin color is of-ten not raised in cross-racial treatment. I was able to raise this topic with Mike and his parents, and the parents could share their above-noted reactions and fears of Mike's selecting a feminine sexual iden-tity, as related to his color and sense of self. Mike initially denied not only his blackness but the reality of our racial differences, telling me that I was the same color as he and his mom were (or even darker, when I tanned over the summers). Over and beyond his initial de-nial of the interracial dyad was, I believe, Mike's need for merger and oneness in his need for me to serve as a selfobject. Over time in the treatment, Mike often stated that it was easier to talk about skin color and race with me than with his family or with any of the black teachers he came to like as his academic success evolved, since I would not get "personally insulted, enraged, or swept away" by his ambivalence about his African American identity. "You don't go off on me, hysterical and furious, when I say that Martin Luther King wasn't the greatest man who ever lived." Mike came to see that over and beyond issues of race were his provocativeness and his passive–aggressive, sly manner of defying and attacking adults. We could ef-fectively engage in what Thompson (1996, p. 125) has called "racial surgery"—namely, helping Mike see the difference between struggles that would be his regardless of ethnicity, and those that were compli-cated because of his race and color.

I concur with Thompson (1996) that in the treatment dyad the affective component of race is a powerful and "unique treatment variable, because of the sheer enormity of its ongoing impact on the reality of African-American patients. . . . Race is a legitimate and necessary aspect of the psychoanalytic exploration for most patients in this culture, but it is so especially for those whose ethnic group define race as an integral part of self-identity" (p. 139). Thus I could not allow it to be bypassed and ignored in my work with Mike and his parents. I believe we were all successful in the psychoanalytic task of exploring this painful and complex issue with the same intensity and clarity that were applied to other aspects of personality in the analytic work.

At the end of treatment, along with enormous gains in all aspects of his life, Mike achieved an "integrative awareness of racial identity"; this is defined by Sue and Sue (1999) as having acquired an inner sense of security regarding self-identity. This was evident in his acquiring pride in his racial heritage, which enabled him to exercise a high degree of creativity, personal freedom, and autonomy. Mike's appreciation for both the white and black races increased as he became more multicultural. No longer frightened by discrimination or oppression from whites or blacks, Mike had better self-esteem, and this included an appreciation of his psychological and intellectual resources to deal with whatever he might encounter. I link his improved racial identity to his similarly attained firm masculine sexual position. The goal of all treatment interventions is the development of a cohesive self (Kohut, 1971).

Countertransferentially, it was often a struggle at first not to censor and exhort Mike to make behavioral changes. Although his regressions and defenses were often exhausting and anxiety-producing, I concentrated on focusing on Mike's subjective inner reality. I attempted to be an inner observer—that is, to use vicarious introspection to gain access to Mike's core of pain, shame, and poor self-esteem, and to the symptoms of disturbance in his sense of self (Lichtenberg, 1983). I could detect feelings of being depleted, weakened, fragmented, helpless, and hopeless underneath Mike's grandiosity, antiblack proclamations, and arrogant withholding at home, at school, and at times in the therapy hour. I often experienced alarm and anxiety about what Mike provoked from peers and teachers. At times I had to calm my sense of urgency when his behaviors caused others to attack and/or abuse him, especially on the playground or in the classroom. I had to frequently remind myself that "treatment of self-disorders requires an extremely slow pace" (Solomon, 1991, p. 130). In line with the research indicating that countertransference dilemmas are greatest with patients who act out or who are highly narcissistic, thereby taxing, provoking, and immobilizing therapists (as well as teachers and parents, when the patients are children), I struggled with and successfully contained any and all impulses to counterattack, lecture, or scold Mike.

Ultimately I experienced profound personal and professional gratification from the excellent progress made by both Mike and his parents. It was thrilling to see this regressed child move forward and more than master age-appropriate tasks. It was equally moving to see the changes in his demeanor—especially his surrender of arrogance, provocativeness, and excessive caution, so that he could be free and spontaneous. Subsequently, our laughter together became a source of mutual pleasure and delight. Anna Freud (1951) noted that therapy cannot be only hard work. She concluded that since child patients rarely come in independently, they require wooing and the establishment of rapport via the use of toys and play within the therapeutic relationship. "In this play world, [a child] is able to carry out actions which, in the real world, remain confined to a fantasy existence" (p. 117).

Moreover, as I have noted elsewhere, "an individualized personalized history empathically understood by the therapist is the key to comprehending what lurks beneath the surface. Obtaining it requires the provision of a compassionate and personal relationship that demonstrates mutuality, concern, and feeling a genuine relatedness towards the patient" (Mishne, 1996, p. 151). According to Guntrip (1975), to find a good parent at the start is the basis of psychic health. If a good parent is lacking, to find a genuine good object as one's therapist is both a transference experience and a real-life experience. I often wondered about the ingredients of the good object—me, for Mike and his parents; and Mike's parents' becoming that, for him and for each other.

Atwood and Stolorow (1984) define psychoanalysis as an intersubjective science, focused on the interplay between the differently organized subjective worlds of the observer and the observed. "The observational stance is always one within, rather than outside, the intersubjective field. Psychoanalysis is unique among the sciences in that the observer is also the observed" (pp. 41–42). In another publication, these authors posit that the intersubjective approach greatly facilitates empathic access to the patient's subjective world, and that "the only reality relevant and accessible to psychoanalytic inquiry (that is, to empathy and introspection) is subjective reality, that of the patient, that of the analyst, and the psychological field created by the interplay between the two" (Stolorow, Brandchaft, & Atwood, 1987, p. 4).

In attempting to explain the success in the treatment of Mike and his parents, I often pondered the elements of what always felt like a most positive fit between the members of the family and myself. Whereas I was clear about my observations of them, I wondered about their subjective reality experience of me. Although my life experiences did not match Mike's and his parents' lives, I believe that I always could understand and accept their respective values, world views, and concerns. My comfort level with this child and his parents was based in part, I believe, on my fund of specific knowledge and information about African American working- and middle-class urban families. As I have noted in Chapters 3 and 4, I had had extensive experience in treating black clients and in working with black professional colleagues; I also enjoy significant, lengthy intimate relationships with several close black friends. In addition to my awareness of my own cultural and ethnic heritage, I believe I was aware of my own values and biases. I think that Mike and his parents sensed my comfort with them, as well as my respect for their motivation, psychological-mindedness, impressive intellect, and commitment to treatment. Our shared values about help seeking, family ties, educational goals, music, and other topics were, I believe, mutually apparent. I believe that the parents recognized my cognizance of the impact of racism on them; it had hampered what had been their original educational and career aspirations. I also believe the parents recognized my understanding of their lifelong financial deprivation and economic stress, as noted earlier. The parents did not experience being pitied as individuals with endless deficits; rather, I believe they perceived and experienced my respect for their strengths, and their efforts and successes in maintenance of family life.

Because of my long-standing familiarity with African American clients, colleagues, and close friends, I was also immediately aware of the conspicuous role skin color played in this family and for Mike. I had no a priori assumptions about Mike's light color, or about his and his parents' response to it. My prior personal and professional contacts and experiences all had borne out Thompson's (1996) reflections: "The significance of color is surely not unidirectional. While light skin may be valued in many families, in some it is dark skin that is prized. In yet other families, color is truly irrelevant" (p. 127). The family and I enjoyed our special rapport in large measure, I believe, because of the total absence of stereotypes on all of our parts. A. C. Jones (1985) points out the "enormous within-group variability" in the black community; obviously the same variability exists in the white community. I believe that the family perceived my comfort with what Falicov (1998) calls the "ever-present double discourse"—an ability to see the shared human qualities that link us beyond class, color, ethnicity, and gender, while at the same time acknowledging and respecting culture-specific differences that exist because of these factors.

I conclude by pondering my present countertransference response to this child and his parents, who were treated quite some time ago. Success in the work accomplished with a most interesting child is, in part, what compelled me to include this case in this text. In addition, I wish to refute the racist, biased questions that continue to be raised about the value of psychodynamically oriented therapies with minority patients, who supposedly lack the ability to explore the meaning of their experiences (Olarte & Lenz, 1984). Such stereotyping chronically enrages me. Alongside my pleasure in reviewing the therapy with Mike and his parents, I realize that every time I think about this family, I am also dealing with my anger and sense of injustice about the paucity of similar long-term intensive treatment for ethnically diverse patient populations, and especially for all clients of color seeking and needing clinical services. For far too long, such clients have been mythologized as untreatable, and/or totally incapable of using intensive insight-oriented psychotherapy.

It is my contention that this case clearly refutes any and all possible rationalizations about lack of intelligence, capacity for insight, or psychological-mindedness among clients of color—rationalizations that have been offered to explain lack of therapeutic engagement and/or premature termination rates. I would like to demystify the supposed problems and the process of successful long-term analytically oriented work with clients of color. This lengthy case vignette, I hope, illustrates the strength and power of a positive treatment relationship in a cross-racial therapy dyad.

PART IV

The End Phase of the Treatment Process

CHAPTER EIGHT

Working Through

WORKING THROUGH: DEFINITIONS AND CHARACTERISTICS

The term "working through" was originally used by Freud to describe the continuing application of analytic work to overcome resistance persisting after the initial interpretation of repressed instinctual impulses. A later definition is the following: "It is the goal of *working through* to make insight effective, for example, to bring about significant and lasting changes in the patient. Despite initial improvements, unless these traumatic events are thoroughly worked through, therapeutic change will not be maintained and the patient will relapse" (Moore & Fine, 1968, p. 95; emphasis in original). In treatment, patients present such material as moods, affects, symptoms, defenses, stories, daydreams, night dreams, fantasies, hopes, memories, complaints, fears, and activities. Commonly, situations and relationships are described and/or reenacted, whether in the transference proper or in the patient's habitual way of being (a subtype of transference common with children and adolescents, as well as pre-Oedipally arrested adults; see Chapter 5). By following the patient's lead in regard to choice of material and mode of presentation, the therapist can sense how much to reflect and interpret at any given point in the treatment process. Confrontation may be useful on occasion; it can also be nonproductive and in fact assaultive, causing the erection of defenses and resistance, and creating a power struggle and possibly a therapeutic impasse. Active empathic listening is essential, and this precludes the classic paradigm of the "blank screen" therapist. It also precludes any prolonged silences in treatment, which commonly mobilize projective mechanisms, anxiety, acting out, withdrawal, or negativism. It was Blos (1983) who first noted the disorganizing influences of silences.

A therapist often wonders about trying to understand everything at once, and about the optimal timing for interpretations and reflections that will enhance and facilitate the process of working through. Edward (1996) notes that models of the mind and other theories influence how therapists listen to patients. Clinicians must have theories to orient and direct their listening, their interpretations of what they have heard, and their subsequent interventions. These theories serve as a structure that helps to direct and hold us as therapists (Casement, 1990). According to Sanville (1987), we cannot function as clinicians without theory, but it should guide us rather than constrict us in understanding our patients. Practice wisdom has shown that significant activities, affects, fears, and relationships will reappear repeatedly and cannot be handled when initially recognized. Many clients will stop talking if interpretations are too quick and direct, bringing the clients too rapidly into contact with painful material—especially sexual and aggressive material, and feelings of shame and low self-esteem. It is important and indeed "necessary to differentiate between the problem of phrasing an interpretation so that the unconscious and repressed material can be made conscious and acceptable to the patient, on the one hand, and the problem of choosing the right time to give the interpretation to the patient, on the other" (Sandler et al., 1980, pp. 178–179). When a clinician has ascertained what has been expressed, the client may be far from ready to accept the therapist's observation or interpretation. The client's readiness is based on his or her ego state, the nature and strength of the treatment relationship, the current transference and countertransference phenomena, and external factors such as stress and deprivation. The therapist wants to avoid colluding with defenses, such as some clients' propensity to deny and blame others for their current state of stress and turbulence. The process of continual assessment ideally reveals a patient's readiness to hear interpretations (i.e., following mastery of reality and life issues, when acting out and/or self-injurious behaviors are no longer present).

Introspection and insight are linked with working through. Still germane are Sterba's (1934) and Kris's (1956) definitions of these two terms. Sterba described "introspection" as a phenomenon in which one part of the patient's ego identifies with the analyst, shares in the analyst's increased understanding, and takes part in the therapeutic effort. Kris defined "insight" as a process that makes use of the ego function of self-observation in both experiential and reflexive form. Anna Freud (1965) noted that one difference between adult and child patients is that while introspection and insight are normal in adults, they are not present in children: "Children do not scrutinize their thoughts and inner events, at least not unless they are obsessional—that is, to say, in these cases introspection serves pathological rather than constructive ends" (p. 221). Children and many adolescents are not self-observant; rather, they are preoccupied with action and the outer world. However, some teenagers at the time of puberty become excessively introspective as a part of the heightened narcissism inherent in the adolescent process. In general, adolescence proper or middle adolescence is characterized by greater introspection and efforts at self-understanding. Commonly, though, efforts are not directed toward the distant past to comprehend conflict and compulsions to repeat behaviors. Adolescents focus on their current real difficulties and apprehensions about the future. Most commonly, bright, psychologically minded adult patients are the ones who identify with and internalize the analyzing, observing, and reflecting function of their therapists, and who can acquire the understanding of the genesis of their difficulties that is essential to the working-through process.

It is important to bear in mind the limitations of insight. Self-understanding does not produce immediate, magical change and relief. Genuine, in-depth working through and resolution of both internalized and externalized conflict require considerable time, as well as repeated encounters and experience with mastery. For an adolescent, sufficient working through has taken place "when the [young patient] has moved to the next level of development and established himself there" (Sandler et al., 1980, p. 184). With an adult patient, who reflects greater personality consolidation and stabilization, the therapist may anticipate and expect clarity and purposeful actions, predictability, constancy of emotions, stable self-esteem, a consistent value system, and more mature functioning.

From the earliest period in the development of self psychology, Kohut and his followers made a marked departure from the classic emphasis on interpretation and conflict, and focused instead on the underlying deficit. This group of clinicians posited that classic interpretations with the goal of insight and working through commonly create a repetition of the original deprivation and lack of empathy that caused the failure in self-development. They described the essential goal of depth psychology as the rehabilitation and reorganization of the self (Kohut & Wolf, 1978). The self-psychological paradigm emphasizes empathic responsiveness to the patient's needs for admiration and mirroring, as well as the need to idealize the clinician; this warmer approach is contrasted with analytic neutrality carried to the extreme in astute, cold incisiveness.

In treatment, a self-psychological therapist attempts to explain without censure the protective function of the patient's grandiose fantasies and social isolation, in order to demonstrate attunement "with the patient's disintegration, anxiety and shame concerning his precariously established self" (Kohut & Wolf, 1978, p. 421). There is a reconstruction in the treatment of the original self-strivings of the patient, who suffered from uneven or erratic parental admiration or profound disappointment in a parent he or she could not idealize and admire. The therapy permits a "re-examination of the parents' original empathic failures and an opportunity for renewed growth as the patient senses a new object" (Cooper, Frances, & Sacks, 1986, p. 136).

The treatment process relies on techniques of understanding, explanation, and interpretation, with the therapist immersing him- or herself empathically in the patient's demands, hopes, ambitions, struggles, and symptomatic behavior, to gain a more profound emotional understanding of all these. "To put it another way, the theory of self psychology removes the focus from the patient's faulty functioning in favor of learning to understand the underlying structure responsible for the faulty functioning" (Brasch, 1986, p. 409). This approach alters the common classic position of critically confronting the patient's evasions, demands, and actions; rather, the therapeutic goal is structure building, as described in Chapter 5.

"According to self psychology, then, the essence of the psychoanalytic cure resides in the patient's newly acquired ability to seek out appropriate selfobjects, both mirroring and idealizable, as they present themselves in his realistic surroundings and to be sustained by them" (Kohut, 1984, p. 77). In addition, Kohut (1984) considered treatment and working through as completed when there is adequate compensatory structure that allows "the unfolding, the flowering, and the ultimate fruition via creative/productive action of a person's central life program as shaped by his particular ambitions, talents and ideals" (p. 205). This focus on the quality of the patient's life is in contrast to classic goals regarding resolution of conflict, drive modulation, and making the unconscious conscious. A successful cure and the accomplishment of working through emanate from countless repetitions of understanding and explaining, via empathic, nonconfrontative interpretations, what went wrong— interpretations provided without hidden moral and educational pressure.

MANAGED CARE AND MODIFICATION
OF GOALS IN THE END PHASE OF TREATMENT

The impact of managed care has greatly reduced the length of time a patient or client can be a recipient of therapy. This profoundly limits opportunities for working through—in other words, the possibility of achieving insight and significant and lasting changes. (It can also compromise the process of termination or eliminate it altogether; see

Chapter 9.) Short-term models of treatment predate managed care, of course. The most common of these models in mental health practice, according to Goldstein and Noonan (1999), are (1) the psychodynamic model, (2) the crisis intervention model, and (3) the cognitive-behavioral model. Many clinicians and authors state that selective criteria for time-limited psychodynamic psychotherapy include the following: patients' presenting symptoms and problems of a recent nature; ability to engage, to relate, and to sustain object ties with ease; a high degree of motivation; and an overall history of adequate adjustment. Problems considered amenable to brief psychotherapy include various circumscribed problems, transient regressions and reactive disorders, or mild exaggerations of otherwise age-appropriate behaviors. Other criteria are the abilities to develop a working relationship fairly easily; to maintain a focus; to demonstrate basic trust and flexibility; and to respond to interpretations, suggestions, and reflections. An appropriate emotional climate in the home further enhances the possibility of successful short-term treatment.

Among the exclusion criteria for short-term psychodynamic treatment are long-standing, chronic characterological difficulties and ego weakness. Patients with such problems need long-term care and often a range of interventions, such as protection and concrete services, as well as referral to residential facilities and inpatient programs. Object loss, severe deprivation, profound family psychopathology (e.g., domestic violence), substance abuse, and psychotic symptoms all suggest the need for long-term treatment. Individuals with sociopathy, excessive acting out or impulsivity, a lack of motivation, and/or an unwillingness to engage in treatment are also not appropriate candidates for short-term intervention.

Again, because of the brevity of the short-term treatment process, there is usually no attempt to restructure the client's personality or to aim for any working through or permanent change. Rather, the interventions are aimed at "modifying the existing balance of forces, both internal and external to the [client]" (Messer & Warren, 1995, p. 285). Goals include symptom reduction and restoration of equilibrium. The clinical focus is commonly on some apparent, easily identifiable life stressor or family situation, requiring modification to improve coping and to lessen anxiety and stress. Techniques or interventions commonly used are clarification, confrontation, support, reassurance, advice and education, collaboration, referral, and advocacy.

Unfortunately, issues of inclusion and exclusion criteria for short-term treatment are not generally considered. Issues of suitability and of individualized assessment and case planning have been ignored by third-party insurance carriers. Concerns must be articulated as clinicians face "the current trend towards corporatization of psychotherapeutic practice and the large-scale deployment of time-limited psychotherapy models as the only available therapeutic option" (Messer & Warren, 1995, p. 329). Messer and Warren (1995) caution about overly optimistic recommendations for brief therapies even for extremely disturbed patients; by way of explanation, they cite the countertransference of grandiosity, as clinicians long for a sense of competence, effectiveness, efficiency, and control. A second source of therapeutic overoptimism is some clinicians' need to "deny the more painful and unpleasant aspects of the human experience by minimizing emotional suffering. It is all too easy to accept our patients' superficial solutions to life's experience because it makes our jobs easier" (Messer & Warren, 1995, p. 332). Less optimistic clinicians, wearied by the struggles with the managed care industry, simply drop out of affiliation with health maintenance organizations and insurance companies. Anger, silence, avoidance, resentful compliance, and passivity are other widespread responses by clients and clinicians alike to the problematic aspects of individualized treatment planning under the constraints of managed care. If a great many clients are to achieve anything like a thorough cure, the managed care industry will need to reconsider its current attitude toward long-term, insight-oriented treatment aimed at genuine working through.

THE IMPACT OF CULTURAL TRANSFERENCE
AND CULTURAL COUNTERTRANSFERENCE
ON WORKING THROUGH

Throughout this book, I have noted the persistence of biased reservations and questions about the validity of using insight-oriented therapies with minority clients, who supposedly lack the capacity to explore the meaning of their psychological life, motivations, and inner experience (Olarte & Lenz, 1984). Such questions suggest negative cultural countertransference, and forcefully impede and interfere with the evolution of a trusting relationship, an alliance, and any process of working through. In cross-cultural treatment, unacknowledged aspects of the cultural identities of patient and clinician can result in a connection that is not optimally respectful of the patient, and even unconsciously or inadvertently biased or prejudiced (due to unrecognized racism, sexism, homophobia, and/or intolerance based on religion or ethnicity). As I have described in Chapter 5, these cultural, racial, ethnic, and gender-related factors can arouse transference and countertransference responses either when the clinician and the patient are of different ethnicities (an interethnic dyad) or when they share a common ethnicity (an intraethnic dyad).

Comas-Díaz and Jacobsen (1991) describe the enormous range of possibilities that can complicate the treatment process in general and the working-through stage of treatment, where insights and improvements are achieved and sustained, in particular. Problematic interethnic transference reactions include overcompliance and friendliness; denial of ethnicity and culture; and mistrust, suspicion, and hostility (e.g., distrust and fear of a perceived power differential). Sharing the same race and/or ethnicity is no guarantee of easy rapport and empathy. In fact, many minority clients view "their own" as less competent than white middle-class professionals. Conversely, some minority therapists are often hardest on those like them for their dysfunctional lifestyles, or feel guilty about being more privileged; ethnic countertransference can also result in over-identification, anger, cultural myopia, or distancing. Interethnic countertransference can arouse denial of ethnic/cultural differences, guilt, pity, aggression, and ambivalence (Comas-Díaz & Jacobsen, 1991).

Perez Foster (1999) focuses particularly on the therapist's subjective state in the process of cross-cultural clinical work. It is her contention that any therapist working with a client whose class, race, or ethnic group differs from the therapist's own enters that situation with predeveloped strands of cognition and affects about that client, which she terms "clinician's cultural countertransference":

> This is a pre-existing countertransferential set within the therapist's psyche, if you will, that is comprised of a complex matrix of cognitive and affective factors operating on varied levels of consciousness. This matrix includes the clinician's own culturally based life values: academically based theoretical beliefs and clinical practices; emotionally charged prejudices about ethnic groups; and biases about [his or her] own ethnic self-identity. These factors represent the therapist's own particular culture-driven countertransference which can be communicated, or projected onto ethnic clients at multiple levels of interpersonal and intersubjective contact. (p. 270)

Perez Foster contends that every cross-cultural therapeutic dyad contains fears, conflicts, and suspicions that both patient and clinician find difficult or impossible to discuss and examine. Failure to achieve insight into these phenomena and work through them can compromise the treatment or even cause premature termination. Thus, in a two-person psychology further challenged by cross-cultural and cross-racial variables, clinicians "must be able to reflect upon themselves as the objects of their own investigations, and to secure themselves as the objects of the intentions and desires of their patients" (Aron, 1996, quoted in Perez Foster, 1999, p. 272). The perspective of intersubjectivity is particularly well suited to cross-cultural therapy, because of the emphasis on verbal and nonverbal "meeting of minds," to use Aron's (1996) term. This meeting must of course include an appreciation of both the client's and the clinician's cultural identity (including their immigration history, symptom expression, and support system; Lu et al., 1995), but it must go even beyond that.

The intersubjective perspective modifies the traditional concept of transference, seeing it as an instance of "organizing activity, a microcosm of the patient's whole psychological life, and from this perspective is neither a regression to, nor a displacement from, the past, but rather, an expression of the continuing influence of organizing principles and imagery" (Mishne, 1993, p. 406) that evolved out of a patient's early formative years. Stolorow, Brand-chaft, Atwood, and Lachmann (1987) emphasize the psychological process of organizing current experience, to which *both* patient and therapist contribute. According to these authors, the multiple functions of transference (to be worked through) are as follows: (1) fulfilling of cherished wishes and urgent desires; (2) providing moral restraint and self-punishment; (3) assisting in the adaption to difficult realities; (4) maintaining or restoring precarious, disin-tegration-prone self and object images; and (5) defensively warding off configurations of experience that are felt to be conflictual or dangerous.

Thus the task of working through is accomplished by the inter-acting dynamics of the client and clinician, and by the influence they have upon each other. Again, this intersubjective communication goes beyond verbal communication, and ideally modifies and changes what Perez Foster (1999) describes as the inevitable fears, conflicts, and suspicions that both parties experience in the cross-cultural therapeutic dyad. I contend that in cases where genuine working through has occurred, patient and therapist are no longer what Perez Foster calls "ethnic strangers."

As a facilitator of working through, the culturally responsive mental health professional (Sue & Sue, 1999) is aware of and sensi-tive to both his or her own cultural heritage and the client's heritage and world view. Valuing and respecting differences are integral fea-tures of a positive treatment relationship. In addition, the majority clinician is aware of his or her position of white privilege, values, and biases (even racist attitudes) and of how they may affect minor-ity clients. By the end phase of treatment, the culturally responsive clinician will be not only knowledgeable about but deeply attuned to the client's personal history, particular ethnic experiences, cultural values, and lifestyle. As emphasized throughout this book, rapport, communication, and comprehension of a wide variety of verbal and nonverbal responses are inherent in a sensitive and empathic rela-tionship.

CASE OF EVA: EXAMPLE OF THE POTENTIAL FOR WORKING THROUGH IN THE ASSESSMENT AND TREATMENT OF A CARIBBEAN-BORN WOMAN OF COLOR

Background and Assessment Information*

HISTORY OF PRESENTING COMPLAINTS

Eva's original presenting complaint was the depression that followed the breakup of a lengthy relationship approximately 5 months before she sought treatment. She had been involved with a fellow graduate student for 4 years, during the last of which they lived together. When Eva and Bill originally met, Bill was still legally married but separated, and the friendship that began in school evolved into a love relationship. Their natural closeness, very good communication, intellectual stimulation, and excitement were the attractions, but because this man was white, the relationship proved to be most difficult and stressful for Eva. She described Bill as less troubled than she was by their racial differences, given his seeming obliviousness or indifference to public responses. His parents, however, were most disapproving, and his mother was said to have refused to meet her. His father was described as polite, though troubled by their relationship. Bill was said not to be swayed by his parents or by the racial difference; in fact, since the breakup with Eva, he had become involved with another black woman (Eva's former friend).

Eva's romantic disappointment and pain were not her only presenting complaints. She also described bouts of frightening nightmares. One recurrent one was a dream of being locked in. She would awaken shaking, upset, and frightened, and then would withdraw, unable to share her fright or talk to Bill about her panic and the ensuing sense of alarm. In fact, she had never been able to talk about her bad dreams, and at the time of seeking treatment, she described a new recurrent one about being scolded and criticized. Upon awak-

---

*The organization of this section follows the Hampstead Profile for the Adult Patient (A. Freud, Nagera, & Freud, 1965).

ening, she'd go blank, feel anxiety (e.g., palpitations, panic, butter-flies in her stomach), and find it hard to get out of bed. She would force herself to try to exercise before bathing, dressing, and departing for work. In the course of her turbulent dreams, she'd frequently scratch her chest, breasts, and neck, as though she were choking and clawing for air, and/or fighting off an unseen menacing figure.

DESCRIPTION OF THE PATIENT

Age 35 at the time she first sought therapy with me, Eva was a tall, stately black woman who radiated inordinate presence, intelligence, charm, and wit. She had a definite personal style, which was especially marked when she bothered to take normal pains with her appearance. She was a most accomplished professional engaged in administrative positions in research and social service settings. When we first began therapy, she was employed at a public interest agency, evaluating public policy and various social programs. She also acted as a researcher/consultant and was effective in conducting studies, obtaining grants, and the like.

Being 35 years old, and thus aware of the "biological clock" and her waning childbearing years, Eva felt compelled to make this personal treatment investment in attempting to improve her personal life. She experienced sadness and a lack of energy and enthusiasm about her work and her friends. A number of her friends had married and moved out of the city, and she recognized the growing constriction of her social circle. She often gave in to moods and apathy, and could be listless and depressed, despite acquiring the "dream job" of her career. (Shortly after beginning the job described above, she was offered and took something more to her liking: namely, a high-level administrative position at a community-based agency offering a myriad of services and artistic programs. The art gallery and theater program were of special interest to Eva, and she enjoyed her work, albeit amid routine administrative/political struggles within the agency.)

Eva's personal and professional achievements were considerable, but they no longer provided her unqualified pleasure. Rather, at times she felt a sense of estrangement; this was reminiscent of her entire childhood, when her and her siblings' accomplishments set them apart from all of their peers. As a native of a Caribbean island, she spoke of cultural differences and barriers between her and American blacks, given their different struggles, heritages, and ethnic customs. Because of her intellectual curiosity, voracious reading, and sophisticated knowledge of the arts and literature, she felt at odds with her current peers; they were put off by her forays to museums, her reading of Henry James and other challenging authors, her book- and print-filled apartment, and her general level of intellectual interests and discourse. She and several of her similarly well-educated sisters sometimes commiserated on the good and bad fortune of their upbringing.

FAMILY BACKGROUND

Eva's background was most unusual in that, amidst considerable economic and familial stress, she and her siblings all demonstrated extreme intelligence and perseverance and thereby were accomplished, highly educated, and productive. Personal relationships were more problematic, and Eva reported that she and her two sisters closest in age had been the most severely affected by their parents' marital strife. Eva grew up in Barbuda, an island north of Antigua in the West Indies (the two islands together now form the independent nation of Antigua and Barbuda). She was the 8th of 12 children. Her father was a merchant, and her mother, devoutly religious, was at home full time—raising the 12 children with an iron hand, and often additionally parenting their adolescent friends, who gravitated to the household for days and weeks on end.

The oldest child, a daughter, was educated on scholarships at a prestigious university in Europe. She was employed as a Caribbean development specialist. The next two siblings had less formal education; a brother worked as a manager of a hotel, and a sister worked as a lab technician. Another brother, with a master's degree in math, specialized in computer systems and worked for the United Nations.

Yet another brother was an economics professor at an outstanding university in California, and had several private business ventures in collaboration with other brothers. A sister was an accountant employed by a women's advocacy group, and another brother was a salesman selling medical equipment to hospitals. Still another sister graduated from a top law school and had just moved back to Barbuda. Eva's youngest sister was completing medical school on a full scholarship at a prestigious American university. Eva herself attended a city university for her undergraduate work and a private university school of public policy for her graduate studies, completely supported by scholarships throughout.

Eva had great respect and regard for her mother, whom she described as something of a charismatic character. The mother was devout, yet aware that some of her children were less than observant (in fact, in the case of Eva, totally estranged from any and all religious practices). The mother was also described as oblivious to the reality that the family was very poor, since no matter what, she was determined that they all become educated and accomplished. The siblings grew up in a close, loyal family, and frequently called upon one another for financial supports to complete their education.

Eva said that her parents were at odds on every score. They were not in accord regarding child rearing or religious observances, and presumably her father resented his wife's absorption in the church and in each and every child. The father had died a few years ago, and Eva harbored much guilt over her lack of rapprochement and reconciliation with him. The father was described as a "playboy," given to showering a string of mistresses with his time and money. His adulterous lifestyle was said to be fairly typical and more or less accepted in Caribbean society, but Eva's mother fought and resisted it, and there were many separations and reconciliations between the parents. During Eva's early adolescence, her father was in and out of the family home, giving less and less attention to the younger children, but all the while expecting labor and help from his children in his shop. Often the children, particularly Eva, were used as go-betweens by the parents—transmitting messages, bringing money home to their mother, and generally triangulated between the parents. When

Eva was 15, her mother did an unprecedented thing in Barbuda society: She denounced her husband, dismissed his protestations of caring for her, refused to submit to his style of "marriage plus mistresses," and left home to join her older siblings residing in the United States. While people in Barbuda were amazed by this stunning act, Eva's mother was firm in her resolve to reside apart from her husband. Despite his fury, she simply stayed away, turning over child rearing to her oldest children. The youngest child (then age 10, now in medical school) was taken in by the oldest child; Eva and the sister next to her remained in the family home, cared for by a woman the mother hired from her church. The father was enraged, moved home, dismissed the help, and "suddenly, briefly, was a full-time father." Eva described this period as a most unhappy one, which ended when she was 16 and left home. The sister residing with her was brought to the United States by the mother. Eva and the youngest sister moved into the home of an older married sibling, where she remained until age 20, when she moved to the United States to attend college.

Childhood memories of bad dreams were shared by Eva, who attributed them to the disorganization and strife that always followed the father's recurrent returns to the family home. His explosive temper and meanness, "even to animals," were cited as causing her fearfulness. The father's eruptions were challenged by the older children, who were protective of and aligned with their mother. In attempts to be "objective," Eva acknowledged the mother's provoking the father by her teetotaler/moralist stance, her absorption in her children, and her possible neglect of her husband.

SIGNIFICANT ENVIRONMENTAL CIRCUMSTANCES

Eva clearly acknowledged her childhood and her familial and cultural experiences as having major influences on her development and maturation. Although she presented herself as somewhat rebellious and a "free thinker," the spokesperson for the younger children in the family, she also complied with the overriding family theme of educational achievement and professional success. However, the lack of consistent parenting during her adolescence, coupled with the stresses of immigration during late adolescence, took their toll on her and the other siblings similarly affected by parental loss and the total breakup of the family when the mother left these children and moved to the United States. Eva and the two sisters closest in age to her all became exceptionally well educated, professionally trained, and successful, but were stunted in their personal lives— ineffectual (in contrast to their older siblings) in making durable romantic attachments and marriages. As noted earlier, Eva's initial referral of herself was precipitated by the breakup of the longest relationship she had ever had, which had initially seemed to offer the prospect of marriage.

Loss, abandonment, and resultant depression seemed to characterize Eva's recurrent self-referrals for therapy. While still in school, she had had some therapeutic contact with a social worker counselor at the college. Both of the two times she sought therapy with me, there appeared to be precipitants in the form of losses—not only romantic relationships that ended, but the loss of significant friends and a sibling who no longer resided in the city.

ASSESSMENT OF DRIVE AND EGO–SUPEREGO POSITIONS

A. *The Drivers: Libido*
   a. *Libidinal Position*

Eva had reached an adult heterosexual position, characterized, I think, by unresolved Oedipal configurations and themes. Given her account of her father, he was apparently an ambivalently loved early object, coming and going throughout her life—erratically loving, but also distant, preoccupied, elusive, and at times angry and frightening to her. I would speculate on her never having had a genuinely conflict-free passionate attachment to him. Thus she repeated this pattern in later object finding, consistently "selecting" insecure relationships with men who were elusive, ambivalent, and preoccupied (in at least two instances, with unresolved first marriages).

b. Libido Distribution
1. Cathexis of the Self

Cathexis of the self was uneven. Eva's professional, intellectual, and personal accomplishments did not provide her with consistent satisfaction; in fact, at times she denigrated them because of the sense of emptiness in her personal life. Eva's weight control, exercise, grooming, and care of her apartment all slipped when she felt low self-esteem. At times she briefly held a stance of arrogance and intellectual combativeness, which presumably masked insecurity and uneven regulation of primary and secondary narcissism.

2. Cathexis of Objects

Eva demonstrated having separated and individuated (albeit with some stress) from the primary dyadic relationship with her mother. She could tolerate ambivalence (i.e., good and bad feelings toward her mother), and in all she maintained a positive rapport with her mother. Self and object constancy were demonstrated by the relationship with her mother and by her stable self-definitions, ethics, values, and morals, despite the strains of immigration and necessary cultural assimilation in the United States. She was acutely stressed by a prior transracial romantic relationship, but this in no way lessened her sense of identity as a black person. Similarly, she retained her ethnic connections with the Caribbean, via her involvement with a Caribbean arts and theater group. She appeared arrested in the early Oedipal stage of attachment to her father, demonstrated by replicating the strains of their relationship in subsequent object choices.

c. Aggression

Eva's aggression was not 100% under control. It could be excessively expressed in her sexual/romantic relationships and, on occasions, in her work life. Soon after the beginning of her therapy with me, her self-controls at work were firmly reestablished; given the absence of a romantic tie, aggression was now turned against the self via manifest depression. It also appeared to be a dominant theme in her dream life: aggression directed at herself, most recently in the form of hearing herself scolded and criticized. Associations to recent dreams suggested her own inner voice severely reprimanding her, in much the same fashion as her mother had scolded and reprimanded Eva and all her siblings in childhood. Such defenses as intellectualization and sublimation via artistic and intellectual pursuits were weakening in their capacity to help her bind in anxiety, depression, and aggression.

B. Ego and Superego

There were no signs of deficits in Eva's ego apparatus. There were no basic impairments of perception, memory, or motility, though when she was depressed she experienced slowing down, inertia, and lack of energy to handle work and self-care efficiently. Her ego functions were intact, and her reality testing, speech, and secondary thought processes were all appropriate, strengthened by sensitive self-observation and an observing ego. Danger and depression appeared to emanate from the external world, in the paucity of satisfying relationships; from the id, with its unsatisfied sexual longings; and from the superego, which scolded and chastised her. The customary higher-order defenses were not as effective as they had previously been in maintaining equilibrium. Thus there was resultant symptom formation, particularly depression. The stable and relatively mature superego, which was aim- and direction-giving, appeared critical, marked by a high degree of secondary sexual and aggressive involvement; this resulted in a degree of melancholia the time Eva first presented for treatment with me.

C. Reaction of the Total Personality to Specific Life Situations, Demands, Tasks, and Opportunities

Eva had marked success in all educational and professional activities, as well as her involvement in community activities. However, her habitual capacity for enjoying social companionship and personal relationships seemed impaired by her disappointment in romantic relationships. The plight of well-educated older professional women, especially minority women, has been well documented in recent sociological studies emphasizing the shrinking marriage market for such women (Bell, 1990; Comas-Díaz & Greene, 1994b; McGrath, Keita, Strickland, & Russo, 1990; Watts-Jones, 1980). Eva appeared more vulnerable and less able to withstand disappointments in failed/unsatisfactory relationships than in the past; she was turning inward, bored and ungratified by prior customary activities and social exchanges.

ASSESSMENT OF FIXATION POINTS AND REGRESSIONS

Fixation in the early Oedipal stage was apparent in Eva's ruminations about her deceased father (especially her failure to make peace with him prior to his death), and her similar ruminations about and obsessive review of the last romantic relationship with a similarly erratic, unavailable partner. Her pattern of choosing men who were still married, albeit estranged from their wives, appeared to repeat a fixation on the early Oedipal object—her father, who was married but estranged repeatedly from her mother.

ASSESSMENT OF CONFLICTS

Despite Eva's intellectual insights, she remained strikingly vulnerable and responsive to overtures from less than available men. Her disapproval of these choices appeared to be the theme of her recurrent bad dreams, in which she was threatened, scolded, and punished. She suffered from internalized conflicts, with resultant disharmonies between instinctual wishes and external demands. These conflicts appeared to be manifested in incompatible drive representations, exemplified by unresolved ambivalence, activity, and aggressiveness, versus appropriate calm and inaction. This was something she had become aware of at work, and she was trying to modify her aggressiveness toward her program director.

Treatment (Including a Discussion of Ethnic/ Cultural/Racial Issues)

During Eva's first course of treatment with me, we worked together approximately a year and a half, and real progress was made. Her nightmares gradually subsided and ultimately ceased. She felt less depressed and anxious, more energetic, and more in command of her life, so that she was able to make a positive job change shortly after beginning treatment (see "Description of the Patient," above). She was also able to move on from the relationship with Bill, mourn the broken romantic tie, and connect with a new man—a black colleague at work. But, as Bill had been, this new man was still legally married and heavily embroiled with his estranged wife (in matters pertaining to separation, divorce, and planning for their preschool child). He was erratic, withholding, and ambivalent in sustaining the intense personal intimacy established with Eva. The reality that many women of color are more educated and have better jobs than men of color further aggravated Eva's romantic dilemmas (Comas-Díaz & Greene, 1994b) and caused her to tolerate a frustrating relationship far longer than she would have preferred.

Comas-Díaz (1994) raises the question of how empathic a therapist can be in an interethnic dyad without having experienced the client's ethnic/cultural (or gender-related) reality. She suggests that within "the cross-cultural encounter, clinicians may be able to empathize at a cognitive level, but not necessarily at an affective level. In cognitive empathy therapists can study the client's culture and confer with colleagues who share the client's cultural background" (p. 294). Kleinman's (1989) concept of "empathic witnessing" is appropriate here: A clinician who recognizes his or her ignorance of the client's ethnic/cultural reality can affirm, through such witnessing, the client's experience of this reality.

Indeed, I had not experienced Eva's racial/ethnic/cultural reality or her family environment. Her experiences included membership in an enormous Caribbean family and in a specific fundamentalist religion; parental strife and separation; and upheaval and immigration to the United States. Eva's narrative or life story addressed both the development of her personal identity and her "cultural story," which refers to an ethnic/cultural group's origins, migration, and identity. McGill (1992) suggests that a cultural story is a collective story of coping with life and responses to pain and problems. In accord with Sue and Sue (1999), I could listen and become engrossed in and sensitive to Eva's account of her cultural heritage and world view. I've had much experience in prior clinical work with American-born black women clients, but Eva was my first Caribbean-born black patient. It was fascinating to learn about her life in Barbuda, a colonized island dominated by British culture, missionaries, and religious groups I had no prior familiarity with (e.g., Seventh-Day Adventists). Despite limited familial finances and a large family consisting of 12 children, Eva described none of the economic hardship or poverty of same-size families in urban inner city black ghettos in the United States. Her personal dignity appeared to be the natural outgrowth of her family life, her inordinately strong immediate and extended family ties, her mother's astounding power and charisma, and Eva's own superior intellectual endowment. Eva's style and manner were compelling and intense. The achievements of everyone in the family amazed me, and in accord with Stone (1988), the stories we shared defined the unique nature of this family and Eva's place in it. "Discussing family stories involving female protagonists can build and enhance self-esteem among women of color" (Comas-Díaz, 1994, p. 301); in this case, such stories demonstrated the atypical strengths of Eva, her mother, and all her female siblings.

Although our life experiences were very different in general, I did share with Eva some specific similar experiences in adolescence and early adulthood. Like her, I was inordinately attached to specific intellectual and cultural pursuits not shared with my peer group, and I was influenced by parental aspirations and expectations that also were not shared with my peers and their families. We both had a real emotional investment in and attachment to the arts (museums and artists, music and concerts), as well as to literature in general and specific authors (e.g., Henry James was both Eva's and my favorite author). Thus, both affectively and cognitively, I readily resonated to Eva's articulated concerns of some degree of estrangement from peers; her being considered an "uppity black" was rather like some teasing I'd endured, being dubbed an "egghead/intellectual" during adolescence. In fact, Eva's estrangement was more painful than my temporary stance vis-à-vis my peers, since hers persisted and even increased in tandem with her achievements. She could vividly recount and share all of this with me in the context of our very close relationship.

Our therapeutic relationship was best characterized as a strong and powerful one, and successful interventions helped to develop and solidify a positive therapeutic alliance, a positive idealizing transference, and a positive idealizing maternal countertransference. Our rapport and ease were enhanced by the reality that despite our differences in race, class, and culture, Eva was easily considered an ideal client; that is, she was young, attractive, verbal, intelligent, and successful (a so-called "YAVIS" client—Toupin, 1980). Together, too, Eva and I valued diversity and demonstrated a consciousness of the interaction of culture and a capacity for cultural self-assessment (Cross, Bazron, Dennis, & Isaacs, 1989). Her bicultural identity as an American and Caribbean black was clearly necessary for Eva's optimal and positive self-identity, and our shared recognition of this seemed to enhance the relevance of the psychodynamic psychotherapy and the therapeutic relationship (Chin, 1994).

Eva's family of origin had produced an astounding array of successful professional children. Both the male and female siblings excelled academically, and thereby achieved admission to impressive colleges, universities, and graduate school professional programs. It simply was expected in the family, and all of the children met the familial aspiration and became highly educated, with subsequent impressive high-status jobs and positions. This created a well-known paradox for Eva (and her sisters) within the family's ethnic/cultural/racial community: Her Caribbean black community at home, as well as the black community in the United States, regarded her both as a community heroine and as a traitor. Success can cause alienation from one's ethnic and racial community (especially when few are so successful), as well as a sense of responsibility toward those less fortunate in the community of origin (Comas-Díaz & Greene, 1994b; Comas-Díaz & Jacobsen, 1991; Espin, 1994). Eva acknowledged jealousy of my greater freedom to be "typically" successful. She viewed successful, educated professional Jewish women as the norm, and saw me as conforming to my familial, ethnic, and cultural heritage. Eva's and her female siblings' accomplishments generated a common mixture of reactions in her: depression, pride about achievements, and ambivalence over professional success, because the very strengths of self-reliance often lead to difficulties in establishing intimate relationships (McGrath et al., 1990), with resultant loneliness and isolation. Well-educated professional women are said to face an ever-shrinking marriage market (as noted earlier), and this situation is more extreme for professional women of color, because the women's very competence often threatens eligible males' self-esteem. Eva spoke of not needing help in regard to her sense of competence or empowerment. In fact, she felt that her mother's unique feminist self-assertion and ability to leave her marriage, all "unheard of" in the mother's peer and religious community at home, set a standard of empowerment that Eva and her sisters hoped they could maintain. Eva linked her depression primarily to her problematic romantic relationships. She saw the link between this recurrent phenomenon and earlier sorrow about her lack of being fathered and her parents' chronic strife and ultimate separation.

After the first course of treatment concluded, she sent me a follow-up note:

> Dear Judith: How are you? I just wanted to let you know
> the good news. I got the job, Director of Training at the
> [Y] Community Service Center, of all places, and start in
> two weeks. Everything else is pretty much the same. S
> [most recent boyfriend] remains a deep pain in my gut.
> Talk about mistakes! Anyway I am hoping that the new
> job will give me a fresh start; a chance to heal and forget.
> I really miss our sessions terribly. So many times I have
> wanted to call.
>
> Eva

In the next year, Eva did call requesting additional contact. We resumed weekly sessions, during which time Eva focused on the reappearance of nightmares, depression, and estrangement in her personal life, and on her unresolved feelings about the most recent broken romantic relationship. She also examined both her short-term and long-range professional goals and career aspirations. The nightmares waned once more after our sessions began. During this second course of therapy, I explored more deeply than before what Eva's response might be to a referral for a classical 4- or 5-day-a-week analysis. I based these considerations on her age, her strengths, her intelligence, her psychological-mindedness, and the depth of her problems in the realm of repetitive choices of unavailable romantic partners.

My goal was to educate this promising woman in regard to her strengths, as well as the deeply embedded core neurosis, which I felt would be best treated via an uncovering, insight-oriented, structure-changing, intensive treatment approach. The second course of treatment focused on explaining what analysis was as a mode of therapy, and how it differed from psychotherapy. Eva came to see the basis of this treatment recommendation, as well as my belief that she could benefit from it and thereby make needed in-depth changes. As demonstrated in our recent prior work together, when we both worked our hardest and did our best, such changes were not possible to achieve via less intensive treatment.

The need for internal change in regard to the following appeared relevant. The seeming archaic, harsh, early Oedipal superego structure needed analysis of its sources, so that it could be replaced by a more mature, self-tolerant one. In the course of our psychotherapy, Eva's reminiscences of her mother's and the church's chastisements served to lessen her harsh dream life, but a more in-depth treatment seemed required to effect more lasting and complete change. Also, Eva's libido and aggression were bound up in conflicts and symptom formation, and needed to be released for constructive use.

The following characteristics, attitudes, and circumstances seemed to me to suggest Eva's capacity for genuine working through (i.e., for having a positive reaction to analytic therapy). Eva demonstrated insight into the detrimental nature of her pathology, and a desire for help, cure, and relief. Her prior fear of analysis was due to her apprehensions about getting in touch with painful material, as well as about putting all hope into this enterprise. She had previously struggled, succeeded, and been self-reliant in problem solving. She now acknowledged the limits of conscious, rational, self-directed problem solving and was motivated for demanding analytic work. She had a marked capacity for self-observation and self-evaluation. Because of her exceptional intelligence, she was able to conceptualize ideas and feelings and to express them with verbal sophistication and psychological-mindedness. She demonstrated a high level of object relationships, with clear self–other boundaries and distinction. She appeared capable of developing a transference relationship, with a tolerance for the vicissitudes of the inevitable resistance in the course of treatment. She had good frustration tolerance, good impulse control, the capacity to persevere in the face of difficulties, and areas of established sublimation to displace and neutralize her energies. Her capacity for hope and optimism had not been overshadowed by her current experience of depression; thereby she was persuaded to seek analysis, which I viewed as a demonstration of her sense of hope. Although she half-feared one more "accomplishment" as causing her additional estrangement from less aspiring peers (she'd been labeled in childhood as "one of those 'perfect' children," and in adolescence and adulthood as an "uppity black"), she acknowledged she was who she was. Since she couldn't pretend and hide her intelligence, similarly, she couldn't and wouldn't hide her psychological self-awareness and interest in self understanding.

In summary, I viewed Eva as a most promising candidate for analytic work. She was responsible about appointments and fees (which I had scaled down), and now, I thought, was ready to make this commitment for intensive therapeutic work. I anticipated that she would prove to be a challenging client, given her strong personal style and her set of defenses, as well as her striking intelligence and ability to question authority. Any potential therapist would need to be sensitive to and open to learning about the varied ethnic and cultural differences, all of which Eva could share in a rich and meaningful fashion. She viewed herself as having reached a crossroads regarding her professional and interpersonal future, and thus was highly motivated for analytic work.

Eva was accepted at every psychoanalytic institute where she applied as a low-fee training case. At my request, she was assigned an advanced analytic candidate in training.

The referral of Eva for analysis was intended to facilitate the most in-depth, genuine working through—namely, to make insight effective and to bring about significant and lasting change. Despite her insights achieved in, and excellent response to, our psychotherapy and the therapeutic relationship, Eva only experienced symptom reduction (i.e., a significant decline in depression and aggression). Although she felt better, she still could not avoid the repetitive compulsion in her romantic relationships—that is, becoming involved over and over again with someone like her father, who was unavailable, inconsistently attentive, and involved with "other" women. This core conflict was best treated at an unconscious and preconscious level, via the use of dreams, free association, and heavy reliance on transferential material. While psychotherapy had provided considerable relief, it was ineffectual in genuinely altering her basic core conflict. I did not want to possibly compromise Eva's treatment by attempting to convert our psychotherapy context to one of analysis; I felt that beginning an analysis afresh was in her best interests, hard as it was for us both to let go and conclude our relationship.

CHAPTER NINE

Termination

AN OVERVIEW OF TERMINATION

In the clinical literature, the topic of termination has received relatively scant attention. Some believe that the concluding stage of treatment is the one that produces the greatest amount of stress and difficulty, creating problems for both the patient and the clinician. At this point, the affective meaning of the therapy and the significance of the therapist–patient relationship are experienced most keenly— not only by the patient, but also by the therapist (Schiff, 1962).

Orgel (2000), at the fall 1998 meeting of the American Psychoanalytic Association, offered a moving plenary presentation titled "Letting Go: Some Thoughts about Termination." He observed that in the final phase of treatment, he becomes aware of an increase in identifications with his patients:

> Their personal language, bodily attitudes and rhythms, and so on affect my own more strongly during sessions, or at other times my thoughts turn to them, probably reflecting my parallel wish to hold on through my identification with them. These interlocking identifica-

tions, partial and transient, contribute essentially to my attunement to [each patient], and they are intensified in both of us, in the painful hours when loss is anticipated. (p. 731)

He also described patients' oscillating between impulses to hold on firmly and to let go abruptly. Some who have often been late become most punctual; those who never miss sessions suddenly cancel and have absences. Mood shifts are rapid, and during this phase the regressive pull often exerts the greatest pressure on the analyst.

How the therapeutic relationship is brought to a conclusion may in fact be the most important aspect of the entire treatment process, in that it generally influences the manner and degree to which gains are maintained. Commonly, failure to work through the attitudes and feelings related to the ending of therapy will result in a weakening or undoing of the therapeutic work.

The paucity of writings on this topic in the clinical literature has been attributed to the reality that saying goodbye is hard, "often as difficult for the worker as for the client" (Gutheil, 1993, p. 164). Termination rekindles both clients' and clinicians' feelings about prior separations and losses (Germain & Gitterman, 1980; Hepworth & Larson, 1986; Webb, 1985). Gutheil (1993) observes that termination may spark feelings of guilt in workers who regret not having done more for their clients. Kohrman (1969) observes that therapists have particular difficulty in separating from and relinquishing younger patients (i.e., children and adolescents), which undoubtedly reflects their attitudes and anxieties about surrendering the parental hope of safeguarding the young persons.

Ferenczi (1927/1955) was the first to focus specifically on the concluding phase of treatment; he noted that completion is attainable "only if unlimited time is at one's disposal" (p. 82). The next significant examination was Freud's (1937) seminal paper "Analysis Terminable and Interminable," in which he offered guidelines and criteria for concluding analytic treatment. He emphasized relief of the patient's suffering, the conquering of anxieties and inhibitions, and the therapist's conviction that the treatment has been successful enough to ensure against any repetition of the patient's symptoms and pathology. Freud was not unrealistic in his expectations of treatment gains and goals in considering when appropriately to conclude treatment. He emphasized sufficient intrapsychic structural change to permit optimal functioning. This would be exemplified by the modification of a patient's harsh superego and the diminution of defenses causing secondary interference. The pioneer work of Ferenczi and Freud raised the critical questions clinicians and health care providers still wrestle with in considering when and how to conclude therapeutic interventions. Briefly, they are as follows: What is the age-appropriate functioning that signifies mental health, and what are the criteria for termination of long-term and short-term treatment?

In the 1960s and 1970s, brief or short-term therapy became increasingly recognized as a valid form of treatment—one that provides specific significant help and is not an abbreviated or watered-down, inferior version of open-ended long-term treatment. Mann (1973) raised questions about the "interminability" of open-ended treatment, and suggested that vaguely defined goals and therapists' countertransference problems caused inappropriately prolonged therapy. Some practitioners, such as Maluccio and Marlow (1974), advocated the use of a treatment contract to ensure patient–therapist interaction and collaboration in identifying concerns, goals, conditions of ongoing service, and time allotted for the therapeutic intervention.

Unfortunately, contemporary practice more frequently mandates brief treatment in which patient–therapist collaboration on selection of goals is *not* used as a criterion for determining the timing of treatment termination. Rather, due to the current sociopolitical process in determining clinical practice, such decisions are made by third-party payers and managed care personnel. This poses many difficult ethical, clinical, and political questions and dilemmas, as we witness the "industrialization of psychotherapy taking place outside the traditional areas of scholarship, research and reasoned clinical discourse" (Messer & Warren, 1995, p. 331). Too often of late, prescriptions for short-term treatment are mandated by various managed care programs, which remain oblivious to therapists' clinical assessments and recommendations for long-term care. Messer and Warren (1995) warn against overly optimistic recommendations for brief therapies even for extremely troubled patients, as I have described in Chapter 8. Seemingly, many overzealous advocates of brief therapies may never hear the full extent and nature of their clients' pain and suffering.

THE SIGNIFICANCE OF TERMINATION

Most of the literature dealing with termination has been generated by psychoanalysts. "The accumulated body of knowledge that exists in this field as a result of clinical and observational research highlights the point that issues of separation and attachment are of particular developmental significance" (Cangelosi, 1997, p. 5). Likewise, termination of treatment entails loss and separation. Termination reactivates earlier losses and separations that both patient and therapist have endured. There are inherent limitations based on the personal strengths/attributes and weaknesses/vulnerabilities of each, as well as the individual nature of each treatment relationship and course of treatment.

Loss is seen as inherent in all ego development, however (Grayson, 1970), and Loewald (1962) noted that separation has the significance of emancipation and growth. Buxbaum (1950), DeWald (1967), and Weiss (1972) all compared termination to the normal progression from adolescence to adulthood. Schafer's (1973) examination of the termination phase emphasized the "unspoken promises, expectations, and resistances on the part of both patient and therapist" (p. 140).

CLIENTS' AND CLINICIANS' RESPONSES TO, AND REASONS FOR, TERMINATION

Ideally, with an appropriate, planned termination, the patient will leave therapy feeling strengthened and fortified by the experience of mastering the current loss via the renewed examination and re-experiencing of old separations and possible traumas. Termination can offer an integrating, corrective opportunity to rework and modify prior separation experiences and problems.

Termination can be seen and experienced as a new beginning, a graduation, or even a "ritual marker of accomplishment. Positive reactions experienced by clients include pride, joy, excitement, a sense of autonomy and maturity" (Fortune, Pearlingo, & Rochelle, 1992, p. 171; see also Garland, Jones, & Kolodny, 1973; Martin & Schurtman, 1985; Polombo, 1982; Wayne & Avery, 1979; Webb, 1985). Less positive client reactions include negative ways of avoiding termination, such as nihilistic flight (Garland et al., 1973), regression (Elbow, 1987), and the development of new symptoms (Firestone, 1974, 1978). Shane and Shane's (1984) account of patients' responses to concluding treatment reflects an ambivalent mix of pride and guilt about their achievements in therapy.

Practitioners' strongest positive reactions to termination are pride in their clients' success and pride in their own professional skill in providing effective helping relationships. Less positive responses by clinicians include relief at concluding taxing relationships, nagging guilt and doubts about their professional effectiveness, doubts about clients' progress, and being overwhelmed with the reexperiencing of previous losses (Fortune et al., 1992). In sum, like their patients, clinicians can suffer grief/mourning responses, denial, sadness, anger, and so on.

Of course, the responses of both a client and a clinician to termination will be affected by the circumstances. In particular, if the termination is premature and necessitated by outside constraints (e.g., insurance edicts) or life changes (e.g., illness or a move by either patient or practitioner), this can stimulate a sense of betrayal, abandonment, or disillusionment. "If a therapist refuses to face the reality of either the seriousness of his/her illness or the need to make plans to terminate, it will be doubly difficult for the patient to deal with the unplanned termination" (Levin, 1998, p. 43). Levin (1998) emphasizes the need for the therapist to be authentic and honest and to disclose facts as soon as possible, so that the patient can have options and some sense of control about choices ahead, including grieving for the loss to come.

Siebold (1991) has examined the transference and countertransference issues surrounding her own experience when she moved to another state, requiring transfer of or termination with her patients. She utilizes the concept of an "anticipatory grief reaction" as an additional way to understand and describe a patient's experience of being left. "Although forced termination is a narcissistic wound inflicted by the therapist, the therapist's management of the ending can render the process productive for the patient" (Siebold, 1991, p. 203). Siebold emphasizes anxiety, anger, denial, idealizations, and deidealizations during transfer or termination, as experienced by both client and clinician. In transferred cases, the crucial final actor is the client's new therapist, whose sensitivity and appreciation for the need to mourn can assist a client in the necessary working through and "letting go" inherent in a forced termination. In a subsequent article, Siebold (1992) offers additional reflections on forced terminations and concludes that although such endings are not optimal, they are potential opportunities for maturation, growth, and mastery. Rather than creating only mournful feelings and a process fraught with peril, forced terminations also create opportunities for previously unavailable material to be aroused. With supportive interventions, a client can be assisted to master a forced termination effectively.

In clinical practice with children, premature, unplanned terminations may be initiated by parents, by a child, or by the therapist. Young families tend to move frequently, due to parents' job changes, divorce, remarriage, economic difficulty, or a decision to seek better schools; parental resistance can also provoke an unplanned or even ill-advised conclusion of treatment. Children, like their parents, can become resistive, particularly when faced with some anxiety-provoking and emotionally charged issues. When parents are also resistive, they often accept the children's articulated desire to stop the therapy. In other cases, children feel disloyal to their parents if they find themselves becoming close and intimate with their therapists (Cangelosi, 1997). Unresolved separation/individuation issues can interfere with a child's readiness to connect to another person, and thereby distance him- or herself from the mother. Weiss (1991) also observes that a clinician's problematic countertransference can support or even initiate a premature termination. This may be due to the therapist's difficulty in tolerating the various attitudes, behaviors, and affects a child presents. Finally, as with adult clients, therapists may initiate termination with child clients because of changes in the therapists' personal lives (e.g., job change or relocation, illness, or pregnancy).

Premature but planned terminations commonly occur with all client groups in training settings when interns or students conclude the academic year. Gould (1978) examined the termination of therapy created by the conclusion of social work students' fieldwork placements, psychologists' internships, and psychiatrists' residencies. The trainees interviewed in Gould's study experienced dismay that they were unable to see their work through to completion, and they doubted whether their clients could have had a good experience. There exists considerable controversy about whether or not student clinicians should inform patients from the start of their trainee status and the fact that they will depart 8–9 months later. Some settings still advocate that this reality should be withheld, as it discourages engagement in treatment and the establishment of an alliance, and stimulates separation anxiety. Others differ, noting that the failure to share is a betrayal of trust; as such, it interferes with a trainee's sense of freedom in the treatment relationship, and thereby the ongoing work with the client. Trainees also confess to feeling guilty about "exploitively" learning from their patients. In more recent years, with ever-increasing abbreviated therapy in mental health clinics and social agencies, a trainee's academic year is commonly not an abbreviated course of therapy—although it is often less than adequate for a client, who must repeatedly return and reapply for help in the revolving door of contemporary agency-based practice.

Before the last decade or so, there was a paucity of literature and research regarding issues of clinicians' responses to, or satisfaction with, termination. The subject is currently receiving increased attention, but the major inquiries center on psychoanalytic interventions and long-term counseling settings. (By way of contrast, it should be noted that clinicians engaged in hospital work commonly provide short-term crisis intervention services and seldom have an opportunity to terminate services formally; see below.)

In a relatively recent study, Resnick and Dzieglewski (1996) found that practitioners are more uncomfortable when outcome results and client feedback are unavailable, and there is inadequate opportunity to review interventions and take pride in a job well done. Especially in cases where unplanned terminations occur, there is a "decrease in job satisfaction" (Resnick & Dzieglewski, 1996, p. 30). On the other hand, the authors found that their study supports previous research indicating that clinicians' enjoyment of their professional responsibilities is associated positively with a sense that their work contributes to or benefits their clients. Accordingly, being able to plan termination on the basis of actual, thoughtful goals and objectives, and to receive feedback from patients or families, decreases job stress and increases job satisfaction.

At present, there are various settings in which, by the nature of the services rendered, there is little opportunity to execute a planned formal termination. These settings are often providing emergency/crisis intervention services, largely to clients of color; client feedback is too frequently ignored in these contexts, and outcome results remain ambiguous. Such settings include hospital emergency rooms, victim services, substance abuse programs, HIV/AIDS programs, methadone maintenance programs, child welfare services, and the like. The urban poor, who are continually engaged in a struggle for sheer survival, commonly develop "feelings of marginality, alienation, helplessness, powerlessness and anomie" (Thompson, 1995, p. 534); as a result, they may feel passive in response to any treatment interventions, and the (inappropriate) termination of therapy may be no exception. Cultural racism as a narcissistic trauma that causes its victims to feel perceived as less than human by the social milieu is discussed by Miliora (2000). Such experiences can assault self-esteem and cause a "depression of disenfranchisement" (Miliora, 2000, p. 43). Commonly, the staff members in these settings are marginally trained, undersupervised, and overworked. Because the clients in these settings are generally viewed as unable to utilize psychodynamic therapy, there continue to be marginal commitments to improve services to the urban poor. This perspective (misguided, I believe) is slowly changing, particularly in the child welfare field, where it is recognized that there is an urgent need for better services. I concur with Javier (1996) on the frequent need to make adjustments in traditional *psychoanalytic approaches* when treating a more deprived and disturbed population, while applying *psychoanalytic principles* in unaltered form. I also concur with the recommendations offered by Resnick and Dzieglewski (1996) in regard to improving the handling of termination, increasing job satisfaction among clinicians, and thereby providing better services to clients. These authors point out the benefit of implementing more formal case terminations or discharge plans, followed by pursuit of evaluation and feedback from clients, interdisciplinary colleagues, coworkers, and others, to effect better communication between discharge departments and the community agencies to which clients are referred. Postdischarge case conferring and the above-noted efforts should decrease workers' feelings of social isolation—feelings that are exacerbated by the reality of managed care, which will increase the negative impact of unplanned terminations on job satisfaction (Resnick & Dzieglewski, 1996).

CRITERIA FOR THE APPROPRIATE CONCLUSION OF TREATMENT

General Considerations

The indications for the appropriate conclusion of treatment are many and varied, and require consideration from both ideal and practical standpoints. Most clinicians who are not answerable to managed care companies stress that the decision to end therapy should not be solely based on symptom relief. In discussing termination in work with children and adolescents, Neubauer (1968) recommended a developmental assessment to ascertain whether a young patient demonstrates noteworthy progress, especially movement beyond points of fixation (notwithstanding phase-appropriate conflicts and problems), and whether the young person demonstrates the capability to handle ongoing and predictable future developmental and environmental realities. Anna Freud's (1962) classic criterion is most apt today; she stressed the need to examine drive expression and ego–superego functioning for "signs of age-adequateness, precocity, or retardation" (p. 55). A child's capacity to develop progressively—or, conversely, the damage to that capacity—is the most significant feature in determining the child's mental future. In considering the ideal criteria for termination, however, one must continually return to the process of assessment, since neither symptomatology nor the accomplishment of life tasks alone can serve as the sole reliable guide.

In assessing the readiness for termination in clients of all ages, the clinician attempts to ascertain personal strengths and weaknesses, as well as external familial and environmental circumstances that may enhance or impede future coping and adaptation. In clinical work, common goals include increasing the capacity for reality testing; better coping with and mastery of age- and stage-appropriate roles and tasks; more age-adequate object relationships; and improvements in capacity for work. Self-esteem and self-awareness are other measures or criteria to assess when one is considering termination.

Considerations in Multicultural Practice

In multicultural practice, a clinician needs to be sensitive to the following before considering termination. Optimally clients have achieved, or at least have substantially improved, their racial/ethnic identity development, and are better able to manage the tensions between varied cultural worlds. All clients' cultures are composed of collective identities (Falicov, 1998) that only become reconciled once they have gained acceptance and security in living a bicultural existence. This is a crucial treatment goal in work with minority clients, and can evolve out of a therapeutic relationship that demonstrates respect and positive regard. Sue and Sue (1990) describe this advanced stage as that of "integrative awareness," which can offer "more autonomy, self-esteem, and racial pride" (Cooper & Lesser, 1997, p. 331).

While engaging in cross-racial or cross-cultural therapy, it is essential that issues of race and/or ethnicity be examined and processed. As emphasized throughout this book, color-blindness compromises cross-racial therapy, and so a racially unmatched client and clinician need to examine the effects of race and ethnicity (as well as gender, socioeconomic status, etc.) on the treatment relationship. Clinicians need to add considerations of clients' conflicts with their ethnic/cultural/racial identity as part of a normal developmental struggle to their psychodynamic conceptualizations and formulations about the clients. In treatment dyads where such identity issues and biculturalism are appropriately and emphatically dealt with, there is no conclusive evidence that client–clinician racial differences impair treatment outcome (Cooper & Lesser, 1997; Davis & Procter, 1989). Coleman (2000) reports initial research showing that matching clients and clinicians by ethnicity improved clients' attendance in therapy, but that differences in outcome were not significant.

TECHNIQUES IN TERMINATION

In insight-oriented psychotherapy, the patient and clinician should have successfully resolved the transference relationship, particularly the intensified negative feelings that commonly surface at the loss of a significant relationship. In supportive therapy, the therapist continues attempts to reduce conflict and stress, and avoids mobilization or activation of the negative transference by emphasizing rapport and the positive aspects of the transference. In both circumstances, when possible, the therapist can offer a continuing availability should the patient need it.

In considering the length of time appropriately allocated for termination, a clinician must consider a patient's sensitivity to separation and his or her history of separation traumas; the nature, depth, and length of the treatment relationship; the availability of other persons who might offer support to the patient; and the reasons for the termination. With some clients, especially adolescents, there is an interruption rather than a termination in therapy; teens and some adults take "intermissions" and need to have the security of resumed contact with their therapists upon request. Many settings and professionals can offer a therapeutic stance of flexibility during the concluding stage of treatment.

Ideally, enough time will be allotted to handle the termination. The skilled therapist avoids a narrow interpretation of, for example, the patient's anger, but can also reflect on the patient's sense of loss and sadness. "If the therapist in fact pulls away and detaches himself from the leave-taking experience, the patient becomes abandoned prematurely. [The patient] may now react with mourning and anger. He grieves not for the future anticipated loss of his therapist but for his actual pulling away in the present" (Glenn, 1971, p. 441).

Two extremely important treatment techniques are self-awareness and self-modulation on the part of the clinician, who may be struggling with "overly intense attachment, dislike of the patient, therapeutic over-ambition, or over-identification. Fear of the patient's regression or anger may contaminate an effective termination" (Mishne, 1986, p. 365). A therapist's narcissistic response to the conclusion of therapy can be an important and stressful issue; some clinicians wish to rid themselves quickly of patients who haven't improved fast enough, and/or who haven't made them proud and confident.

Ideally, too, the disposition of every case is well planned, even when a therapist leaves an agency and a case must be prematurely terminated or transferred. In this situation, both patient and therapist will be affected by the termination plan, which may be therapeutically contraindicated (e.g., closing a case despite the need for ongoing care, or placing a case on a lengthy waiting list for eventual reassignment and resumption of care). Such dispositions can elicit feelings of guilt in therapists, who wish they could do more.

THE REAL RELATIONSHIP AT
TERMINATION AND AFTERWARD

Ideally, at the end of treatment the client has accepted the impossibility of obtaining infantile gratifications and has begun to perceive the therapist in a more realistic fashion as transference distortions have begun to resolve. The patient is now experiencing the therapist as a more contemporary real object, and the end of the treatment is viewed as a separation of two individuals who have enjoyed a precious and private collaborative enterprise. Clinicians, especially those in private practice, often receive follow-up letters, pictures, holiday cards, periodic visits, and other updates on their patients' lives. Continued contact or later reconnection with therapists is generally not possible in public agencies and clinics—in part because of logistical factors, and in some settings because continued contact is viewed pejoratively, as due to clinicians' rescue fantasies or need to hold on to patients. Yet if a termination has gone well, a real relationship will have evolved, which can support a client's maintenance of gains and serve as a bridge rather than an obstacle to the future seeking of help (if need be). This "real relationship" must have professional parameters and boundaries in accord with the prior treatment relationship. (Such boundaries preclude friendships, socialization, and/or contact outside the professional office context.)

This experience of the clinician as a real object brings the therapy full circle, back to the early stages of the therapy and the formation of the therapeutic alliance, which is divided into two levels: a rational level and an emotional level. In considering the multicultural alliance, Coleman (2000) suggests that at the rational level, clients from different cultural backgrounds will have different expectations and understandings of psychotherapy and will prefer certain therapist styles. Sue and Zane (1987) consider this working alliance level "credibility," whereby a client feels secure in knowing that the therapist, in the context of a real relationship, is competent and concerned, able to acknowledge cultural differences, and aware of the client's culture. "At the emotional therapeutic alliance level the therapist may be cast into a transference role for which he [is or] is not culturally prepared, and may be confronted with [the therapist's] own conscious and unconscious internalization of racist socialization" (Coleman, 2000, p. 87). The resolution of the emotional part of the multicultural alliance, along with the resolution of transference proper, ideally occurs during the termination stage.

Some agencies and some private practitioners utilize particular termination procedures routinely. These may include an evaluation of the work done together, as well as use of goal attainment scaling, which enables worker and client to examine progress toward specified individualized goals. "Although goal attainment scaling can be helpful at different times during the treatment process, it has special value during termination" (Gutheil, 1993, p. 171). Gutheil (1993), however, cautions on the avoidance of certain pitfalls when termination procedures are integrated into the ending process. Such procedures, like rituals, may take over the attention of patient and therapist, and cut off the expression of emotions and feelings in the final phase. Such termination procedures as formalized evaluations can become a routine part of agency practice, but they should not be used in a rote or perfunctory fashion. Even when such an evaluation procedure demonstrates the achievement of goals, many clients do not want to terminate and end the relationship. It is essential that procedures or rituals not be used to mask or conceal the intense feelings that accompany endings, particularly endings that are forced.

CASE OF JOY: EXAMPLE OF TREATMENT AND TERMINATION WITH AN AFRICAN AMERICAN CHILD AND HER MOTHER

Referral

At age 4½, Joy was referred to my hospital's outpatient children's clinic by her mother, Ms. M, who had previously been a patient in the adult clinic there. The mother, aged 35, an attractive and intelligent African American single parent receiving public assistance, was so overwhelmed by long-standing life problems and by her child that she was contemplating placing Joy in foster care. Ms. M came back to her former therapist to consult about this major decision, and followed his strong recommendation to seek treatment for her child and herself, in order (it was hoped) to avert any need for separation and placement of Joy.

Ms. M's prior therapist and I, who had been assigned to work with her and Joy, shared with each other and the entire clinic professional staff our ample knowledge and misgivings about the local child welfare system. We all were most concerned that if Joy was placed in foster care, she undoubtedly would experience extended and often inappropriate and unnecessary out-of-home placement, and would possibly become lost through "foster care drift." It was also possible that if Joy was placed so young, her mother's legal ties would be terminated, and Joy would not receive prompt adoption services (Morisey, 1990; National Urban League, 1979). All preventative efforts were made to offer services to help this mother and child avoid making use of what we and others (Billingsley & Giovannoni, 1972) view as a failing, racist system:

> Racism manifests itself in the present [child welfare] system of services in three major ways: One, the kinds of services developed are not sufficient to the special situation of Black children. Two, within the system that has developed, Black children are not treated equitably, and Three, efforts to change the system have been incomplete and abortive. (Billingsley & Giovannoni, 1972, p. 28)

Despite the passage of time since this critique was rendered, very little has improved; in fact, because of the high incidence of substance abuse in impoverished black communities, there has been an accompanying rise in poverty among black families. By the mid-1980s, the result was a doubling of the number of black children residing only with their mothers (Children's Defense Fund, 1985), and of those placed in foster care. The rise of HIV/AIDS has only exacerbated this situation further.

An example will illustrate that the problems of serving children and families of color within the child welfare system are made even greater by bureaucratic inefficiency. On March 11,

2001, an article in *The New York Times* (Sengupta, 2001) noted that after 5 years, the cost had more than doubled for the originally planned $113 million computer system intended to improve New York State's long-criticized method of tracking child abuse complaints. The final price tag will possibly be $362 million. In the interim, the Administration for Children's Services has spent (wasted) $15 million more because the system still cannot reliably conduct child abuse background checks, and often confuses the address of the person making a child abuse complaint with that of the person against whom the complaint is lodged. The State of New York has already been fined $3.3 million for its failure to file federally required reports. Problems with the new technology could cause the state to lose $40 million in federal reimbursement (Sengupta, 2001). Such dilemmas in child welfare are commonplace nationally, and demonstrate the validity of the Billingsley and Giovannoni (1972) critique, three decades later.

Assessment of the Mother

In the assessment contacts, the mother's history of victimization was immediately revealed. Ms. M's childhood was a turbulent one due to domestic violence and her father's drinking, which resulted in her parents' divorce when she was 11 years old. Her parents physically fought about her father's drinking, and his jealousy and continual suspicions about his wife. Ms. M and her younger brother were traumatized witnesses, but never endured physical abuse from the father. Ms. M's mother was said to have somewhat decompensated in recent years, as seen in her repetitively poor choices in new romantic partners, since all appeared to be alcoholic and abusive. In addition, Ms. M's mother was moody, at times threatened suicide, and commonly made frightening and dramatic scenes. Ms. M had only meager and marginal contact with her parents and her brother. At age 22 she made a most dysfunctional marriage, which was viewed by her and her prior therapist as replicating many features of her parents' marriage. Since parting from her husband, she had been both a recipient of public assistance and an employee, struggling to make ends meet.

Ms. M and her alcoholic, womanizing husband were married for 9 stress-filled years, marked by terrible fights, separations, and reconciliations. She had five miscarriages prior to the birth of Joy. Mr. and Ms. M had great financial stress, domestic strife, and housing problems (they moved constantly from relatives' homes, to furnished rooms, to hotels, etc.). After their legal separation, they met by accident on the street. Mr. M was apparently suffering a drug- and alcohol-induced psychosis, and he kidnapped his wife, threatening her and Joy's lives as he spoke of voices telling him to kill. In the few intervals when he was not threatening Ms. M, he was begging her to shoot him. Ms. M was almost killed in her escape from this harrowing episode—which followed years of physical and emotional abuse, harassment by her husband's other women, eviction and utility turn-off notices, and a final wrenching separation when Joy was 4 months old. Her overall victimization was both direct and indirect. Pinderhughes (1982) has identified her plight as the victim system of racism and oppression, "where limitations in resources lead to stress, impairments in growth, destabilization of communities and thus more powerlessness. A person who is subjected to a great deal of racist treatment can be afflicted by powerlessness, learned helplessness, depression, and even post-traumatic stress disorder" (Comas-Díaz & Greene, 1994a, p. 343). Hamilton (1989; Hamilton & Jensuold, 1992) also observes defenses like denial in those suffering from posttraumatic stress disorder, which can be revealed by depression, emotional flooding, and disorganized behavior. Her trauma seemingly explained Ms. M's relapsing/regressing into her old conflictual mode of behavior with her daughter, who was now the major target.

I believed that it was crucial to respond immediately and empathically to this overwhelmed mother, since I was very aware of the realities that being subjected to violence can be a serious cause of mental health problems, and that women of color often live in overwhelmingly stressful, antagonistic, even hostile environments (Anderson, 1991). All of these realities were most evident as Ms. M provided the necessary information about Joy's current problems, the child's developmental history, and the above-noted realities of her personal history and significant environmental factors.

Child's History of Presenting Complaints

Ms. M described Joy as having long-standing difficulties: hyperactivity; incessant talking; defiant, provocative, "sassy" behavior; "bossy," hostile interactions with peers and adults; and night fears that caused her to insist on sleeping with her mother. At times when upset, Joy wet her pants by day and/or her bed at night. She was described as always hard to parent, due to colic until she was 10 months old and sleep problems in early infancy. The mother, overwhelmed and exhausted, had frequently let Joy sleep with her since her 18th month (the time of common childhood separation fears). Ms. M recognized that her child mirrored her own overwrought state, as well as the overwhelming marital problems and the parents' separation when Joy was 4 months old. Throughout her marriage, the mother had needed to work; Joy had first been cared for by an inconsistent succession of sitters, and then was placed in a day care nursery at 20 months.

Joy had always been very intellectually advanced, but presently in day care she was commonly "sassy" and sadistic with peers, and thus friendless. She was adult-like in her verbal expression, but also subject to tantrums, continual impatience, and nagging, as she could not wait or tolerate the slightest frustration. Things could and did escalate between the mother and child until the mother exploded and became physically harsh in discipline; Ms. M was fearful of not being able to stop herself from becoming very abusive. Clearly, the mother was frightened as she shared the extent of her anger at her child, but she was also relieved that I did not appear to judge her or threaten her. Instead, I was reassuring that I could and would try to help her with this at once.

Establishing a Therapeutic Alliance with the Mother

Though I was to be Joy's therapist, and Joy's mother was assigned for her own therapy with another clinician (as is usual with children's cases), I intended to have regular, ongoing contact with Ms. M in regard to parent guidance and the development of parenting skills. Thus, in our first meeting I offered her immediate responsive services in regard to her explosive spanking of Joy. I advised her to distance herself from Joy when things became volatile, to allow them both time to calm down. Joy, as expected, refused to stay in her room and/or accept any "time out"; she would follow her mother, torturing, demanding, and also becoming so anxious that she had continual urinary accidents when she and Mommy fought. I then advised Ms. M to get some distance by locking her door for a few minutes, and phoning me whenever things became inflammatory. Obviously I was rarely immediately available at the end of the line, but I would call Ms. M back as soon as possible. She knew she'd never have to wait until the next day to hear from me, and this made her feel supported and not alone. To the best of my ability, I always attempted to offer a respectful, listening ear in an "experience-near" manner; this gave me access to actual events and to Ms. M's emotional experiences, which revealed the core of her pain, shame, and poor self-esteem.

As I have indicated in other chapters, I agree with Chin's (1994) comments that "a therapist cannot begin as a 'blank screen' if he or she is to establish trust and validate the client in a therapeutic alliance" (p. 202). Chin also suggests specifically that a black female client may come to therapy expecting to be blamed, criticized, or put down by a white therapist. Empathizing with clients' feelings regardless of the destructiveness of their behavior is important in all phases of work with maltreated children and their parents, but it is crucial to successful engagement in treatment. A therapeutic alliance results from a client's readiness to accept help and from a worker's ability to mobilize hope, trust, and willingness to work on difficult problems. Thus the worker must make every effort to empathize with parental fears, and needs to convey respect for any positive parental efforts at coping. It is important to move beyond seeing the abused or neglected child as the helpless victim of "bad" parents, to seeing parents also as "victims of their own troubled pasts and current stressors" (Mishne, 1989, p. 45).

Treatment Proper (Including Consideration of Ethnic/Cultural/Racial Issues)

As our work together progressed, Joy's mother was able to share with me what went on at home day by day, hour by hour, and how Joy wore her down with her tantrums. Joy often insisted that her mother take her somewhere after work, no matter what the weather or how tired the mother was. The child seemed to resist being closeted in their small housing project apartment; yet both were locked in a symbiotic relationship that had the flavor of two siblings interacting in a sado-masochistic fashion. When Ms. M was home, Joy would never let her out of her sight; she also insisted that they have the same bedtime, and she refused to close her eyes until her mother went to bed. Ms. M had no life to herself and let Joy accompany her like a peer in their meager social contacts. No privacy was observed in the home. Joy witnessed her mother in the bathroom, and even inside the shower, in their intense dyadic relationship. No relatives served as father surrogates, and the mother received meager support from her own dysfunctional parents, as noted above. Despite all of the mother's overwhelming problems, she was more functional than might be expected, given all of the stressors in her past and current life. Like her brother, she had always maintained employment (even now she was working part time, although she had received public assistance since Joy's birth).

Ms. M's strengths were as discernible as were her vulnerabilities. She demonstrated biculturalism, which Chestang (1979) considers a requirement for blacks. She evidenced the dual perspective of her own family and community system on the one hand, and the larger societal system (with its valuing of education, the arts, and financial independence) on the other. She was most eager to be free of subsidy from public assistance, and was taking some part-time courses in bookkeeping to give her more marketable skills (McAdoo, 1981). Although she was frantic at home with Joy, collapsing into despairing and severe spanking of her child, at her office pictures of Joy were proudly displayed—as were sizeable sums for Joy's "college fund" (a fund the mother initiated and was supported in maintaining by contributions from work colleagues). Despite the mother's commonly feeling at her wits' end with Joy, she envisioned her daughter as an extremely successful adult; to ensure this, she took her very well-dressed daughter weekly to the city museum, children's theater and puppet shows, or the ballet, despite her financial straits. Freeman (1990a) observes that individuals who view themselves as having "missed opportunities" to get ahead in their youth often have high (or even unreasonable) expectations and educational aspirations for their children, once they become parents.

In our discussions of our racial/ethnic differences and what these meant to her, Ms. M repeatedly referred to her own solid black identity. Although she recognized her low self-esteem, she linked this not with race but with class and female subordination (i.e., her mother's abuse by her father, and her own abuse by her husband). She said she wondered at times whether a white professional woman could respect her, considering what she had endured for so long in her abusive marriage. She explained that this was why she had such high hopes for Joy to obtain educational credentials and professional status, and thereby better self-regard than she herself had had to date. The mother volunteered feeling better about herself in tandem with her progress in therapy.

Ms. M differed in numerous ways from many women of color who are victims of domestic violence. Unlike those described by Kanuha (1994), she was not suspicious of mental health practitioners, expecting only to be inadequately served. On the contrary, one of her many strengths was in seeking appropriate resources for help. This was evident in her facilitating a change in her subsidized housing via letters to all officials connected with public housing (including task forces in the mayor's office), as well as in her repeatedly securing long-term psychotherapy for herself and her child in top-notch clinics in her community. She made significant and positive relationships with white clinicians, whom she felt she came to trust in treatment relationships that lasted several years. Despite her lack of formal education, she was very psychologically sophisticated, insightful, and capable of exploring her inner experiences and repetitively painful relationships for the purpose of change.

Diagnostic Assessment of Joy

Joy was a dainty, small-boned, nicely dressed child, with a distinct femininity about her. She was imaginative and most creative in her play, drawings, stories, and enactments. At the time of her evaluation, I assessed her as presenting a narcissistic personality disorder, manifested by poor regulation of self-esteem, grandiosity, and an unusual degree of self-reference. She had significant external conflict with peers, schoolteachers, and her mother. The parents' gross marital problems, and the father's psychotic behavior and financial duress, had created immediate postnatal deprivation and narcissistic injury for Joy. Her mother's need to be employed had prevented early, consistent mothering. Furthermore, the mother's understandably high level of anxiety, plus a paucity of real ties with friends and family, made the mother ambivalently hold onto Joy, preventing her normal separation and individuation. Joy had only partially progressed from dependency to self-reliance in an "as if," precocious fashion. At great cost to herself, she had become proficient at academic learning, but she could not interact with peers or let her mother out of her sight once Ms. M came home from work. She and her mother had endless power struggles over anything and everything, including food, which she handled calmly and normally at school. As noted earlier, bladder control was not consistent, especially when Joy was stressed and/or agitated; however, bowel control had been achieved. Although Joy had not moved much beyond a position of egocentricity in peer relationships, she was able to work actively in nursery school and could learn, produce, and conceptualize in an effective fashion. It was thus concluded that Joy would benefit from analytically oriented psychotherapy.

Reflections on Work with the Mother

Both Ms. M's work with me and her individual psychotherapy sessions enabled her to be very supportive of her daughter's growth and development. Indeed, Joy's progress paralleled her mother's own impressive gains and life changes, which included securing a rent-subsidized apartment (outside the housing project), full-time employment (so that she no longer was a recipient of public assistance), and an adequate income (which enabled her to purchase a long-desired car). Her personal life was expanded via her increased ability to develop and sustain more friendships, as well as a nonabusive romantic relationship.

My work with Ms. M emphasizes what Lichtenberg (1983) has noted as the importance of recognizing "symptomatic alterations in the sense of self, [which include] states of depletion, enfeeblement, a feeling of fragmentation and total helplessness and hopelessness" (p. 170). Self psychology's focus on and attention to impairments in the functioning of the self sensitized me to the mother and child's shared disturbances in self-regulation and the absence of self-soothing and tension regulation. Using the perspective of self psychology, I attempted to employ vicarious introspection and empathy with mother and child alike—as Lichtenberg has recommended, and as I have described in connection with the treatment of Mike and his parents in Chapter 7. Maintaining an empathic vantage point with each family member in such cases requires restraint, careful listening, and hearing the actual pain under the family members' assaultive rage attacks on one another.

Therapy with Joy

Joy was seen twice weekly for a 2-year period, beginning at age 4½. She proved to be of superior intellect, with the ability to draw, play, and create dramatizations and role plays with marked inventiveness. She wrote stories, poetry, and songs, many of which combined fairy tales and children's classic stories with themes from her own life, especially painful loneliness and her longings for an intact family (namely, a daddy and siblings). Joy dictated her stories to me for her story album, a sacred collection we kept in its fancy folder and special drawer in my office for the 2 years we worked together. Examples of her stories and poetry follow:

Jobs

Once upon a time there were some people who had jobs. Some people had no jobs. Mary Poppins had a job. The job was flying with an umbrella. When she was a little girl, she had a mother just like us, and didn't fly. But did her mother bother her!! Then when she grew up she got married and had a baby. She bought a crib for the baby. They had another one. It was a boy. She bought another crib. She had two babies. Then that very day she had another one. The end!! They lived happily ever after.

Babies

Babies grow in people's stomachs. They go into the hospital and sometimes the doctor has to cut the stomach open and get the baby out. My mommy told me when the baby comes out there's a little blood on it, and you have to wash and wipe it off. Babies take bottles which the mommy gets at the hospital store. Some people have boy babies and some have girl babies. The difference is that the girls have more hair. The girl wears girls' shoes and the boy wears boys' shoes.

In recounting this story, Joy suddenly broke into tears, complaining: "Mommy makes all those braids in my hair, and I'm afraid I look like a boy and not a girl. Boys have penises and short hair, and girls have long hair and no penis. Mother couldn't cut it off, I think, so I guess girls never had a penis."

Poem

Once there was a little clown
His name was Tony
The little clown was lonely
One day it was his mother who visited
She had good news saying she is going to the doctor
The doctor said she is expecting a baby
Then the clown shall not be lonely!
The end!
They lived happily ever after.

Using clay, drawing materials, puppets, and a dollhouse and its family of dolls, Joy did many dramatizations and role plays of mother and daughter, or student and nun teacher. She always assumed the adult role, and thus cast me as her daughter, her baby, or her student, to instruct and scold (as seemed to be her reality in the rather authoritarian Catholic parochial school where she attended nursery school and kindergarten). She made construction paper costumes (e.g., hats, purses, and jewelry) to complete her scenarios, for which she composed the scripts, dictating lines for me to record. She was an adorable and engaging youngster, and affection and laughter were major elements of our sessions together over time, as we became more closely related.

Joy manifested acute anxiety at the beginning of treatment. She referred to shots given by doctors, and patients in their beds living at the hospital; these statements reflected her fears that if her mother grew *really* angry, she would carry out her prior threats to give her daughter away, and Joy might be left with me at the hospital. Joy exhibited provocative behaviors in therapy for the first year or more, wanting to rifle through all the drawers in the office, as well as mishandle the phone and drapes. She tried to get me to chase her as she danced about, darting here and there in the clinic lobby and hallways. Simultaneously, she wanted to hit and hug me, to see whether limits would be imposed on her impulses. Her mother, in a poignant tone, repeatedly reflected her relief that Joy acted up with me as well as with her: "I feel such a relief to hear her carrying on with you, like she does with me, because then I feel less guilty, and not totally responsible for her misbehaviors." Joy responded well, though slowly, to being limited with firmness and consistency at home and in my office. She was able to surrender her temper tantrums and attempts to deface and destroy my office. She began to handle frustration in more appropriate ways, mirroring my calm, and thereby gaining in self-regulation and the capacity to soothe and calm herself.

At times Joy wanted to be active, with endless drawings, artistic creations, stories, and imaginative games; at other times, she wanted to be a baby resting in my lap. In the course of the treatment, she idealized me and demonstrated and articulated her wish to be my favorite: "I want to be your favorite of all the kids you see, ever saw, or ever will see!" It proved more fruitful not to puncture or question Joy's grandiosity and need for admiration. She suffered enough at being dressed down at school for similar yearnings. Instead, she was given the admiration and praise she yearned for, and I accepted her need for idealizing me as the therapist.

I made reference to our racial/ethnic differences on occasion, when these seemed possibly pertinent in terms of themes in Joy's play. Her major sentiment seemed to be a dismissal and disavowal of anything that separated us. She often said that there were all kinds of good and bad black people and good and bad white people. Her harsh teacher, Sister Alice, was described as a "bad white lady in her long black dress," and I was referred to as her "good white play lady and special friend." Joy liked the summer months when I'd get a suntan, and she said that after my vacation at "Cape Corn" (Cape Cod), I was tan enough to be mistaken for her mommy or her older sister.

Collaborative Treatment Contacts

Treatment also included regular contact with the mother's therapist and Joy's teachers. School visits were made routinely. I saw Ms. M every 2–3 weeks after the initial period of half a year, when she was seen weekly; I also spoke to her by phone very frequently. Our contact, coupled with Ms. M's own psychotherapy, helped her to become a more consistent, empathic parent, and to understand Joy's alternating adoration and hostility—her idealization and devaluation of her mother, her sole available parent.

Termination Phase

Termination was planned after 2 years of twice-weekly treatment of Joy, and the regular and frequent sessions with the mother described above. The decision to conclude therapy was based on Joy's considerable improvement, as well as the mother's marked gains in effective handling of her daughter; as a result, the emotional tone in the home had changed to one that was well modulated and empathic, and characterized by greater calm, self-control, affection, and humor. Joy's presenting symptoms had lifted. She was no longer enuretic, subject to tantrums, or needing to sleep with her mother. Her stance with her peers and teachers, as well as her mother, was less "bossy" and omnipotent; instead, she had become more age-appropriate in her interactions both at home and at school. Still present, however, were some specific narcissistic modes of relating, characterized by a preoccupation with her own needs and feelings. She was assessed as very bright and doing well at school, though she was seen as performing somewhat under her potential; this was understandable, given the stress she experienced in an overcrowded ghetto inner-city parochial school, which provided after-school day care for children whose parents were employed. A successful referral was made, and Joy was accepted at an excellent private school on scholarship. The termination of treatment was planned many months in advance, taking into account Joy's prior loss of her father, as well as both the mother's and Joy's very strong attachment to me. I also felt strongly bonded and mindful of the stress of "letting go." The mother continued in her own therapy for about half a year following the conclusion of Joy's treatment.

TERMINATION WITH THE MOTHER

Many researcher/clinicians writing about the disparate cultural worlds in cross-cultural treatment stress that therapists must be "aware of reactive arousals, biases and anxieties that emerge within them upon being in the presence of an ethnic stranger" (Perez Foster, 1998a, p. 267). Perez Foster (1998a) and many authors that she cites (Altman, 1995; Javier, 1990; Mays, 1985; Thompson, 1989) posit that cross-cultural, cross-racial, and cross-class clinical interactions are anxiety-laden, and that practitioners are not sufficiently aware of this disavowed and thus unacknowledged cultural countertransference. Perez Foster also focuses on those majority clinicians experienced in working with minority clients who deny ethnic and racial prejudices, and who consider themselves culturally attuned and therefore culturally aware. Although I concur with Perez Foster's perspective and reservations, I also believe that some majority clinicians have had varying levels of experience with different racial and ethnic groups, and that based on their experience (or lack thereof), they react with different degrees of discomfort and anxiety to difficult patient populations.

As I have noted in earlier chapters, I have had lifelong personal experiences and friendships with African Americans. In addition, since I entered graduate training more than half my lifetime ago, I have enjoyed collegial relationships with African American peers, supervisors, and administrators for several decades. I have also treated many children and adults who are African American inner-city urbanites from impoverished backgrounds, as well as a goodly number who are educated, middle-class professionals. Thus I do not view African Americans as "ethnic strangers," as I do other groups with whose members I've had far less familiarity and/or contact. Some specific groups do arouse bias I must face and analyze.

I have always believed in the concept of "fit" between client and clinician, such that some dyads seem to have a special rapport, level of empathy, and depth of understanding, at both the manifest and more latent levels. Nonverbal communication and body language, facial expressions, and eye contact are often avenues of important communication, and so they were between Ms. M and me. Because Joy and her mother remain so vividly etched in my mind's eye, as though our parting was only yesterday, I've long considered and pondered why, and linked these musings to questions about why the work with this child and her mother was so special and pleasurable and the outcome so positive. I attempt to answer these questions in reviewing the feelings and memories of the termination stage.

Although Ms. M was overwhelmed and quite out of control when we began to work together, she was not simply an "acting-out," nonverbal client of color. Quite the contrary: She had had prior treatment, and thus began our contact evidencing considerable self-awareness (albeit without the desired self-control that insight often accompanies). Chin (1994) notes the frequent need for an alternative formulation, to emphasize differences rather than commonality in psychotherapy with women of color. A "difference perspective" would not view differences in psychotherapy as instances of non-compliance and resistance but rather would seek to understand how these differences can contribute to positive adaptations for the client. Therapeutic interventions would be reframed to fit the cultural context; differences would be viewed not as hinderous, but examined for how they might facilitate the psychotherapeutic process. (pp. 206–207)

Thus initially the "hotline" crisis intervention model was offered to Joy's mother, which she used most appropriately until she achieved greater calm and long-desired better self-regulation. This then permitted us (as well as Ms. M and her individual therapist) to work in a more traditional insight-oriented psychodynamic fashion.

Subsequently, in short order, more commonality than expected was apparent—despite the fact that Ms. M was a young single mother of color living in an inner-city housing project, who received public assistance due to meager education and limited job skills, and I was a white Jewish clinician and a middle-aged professor (but also a single parent with one child). Once the mother could contain her aggressive impulses and thoughts, and her tentative plans for placing Joy in foster care, I was increasingly aware of the mounting similarities of my views with her world views. In particular, we shared high aspirations for our children and ourselves.

It was evident that once she was in control, Ms. M all but perfectly met the criteria for what some have defined as an ideal client, the "YAVIS" client (young, attractive, verbal, intelligent, and successful; Toupin, 1980). Though she was not "successful" at the outset of our work, she became so over the course of her treatment, and I experienced much pride and pleasure in sharing her wonder and excitement as she was able to transform her life and thereby also her child's. I was always aware of my initial amazement at her strengths, considering the victimized life she'd endured in her family of origin and in her abusive marriage, as well as the indignities she'd experienced as an impoverished, meagerly educated black woman forced to reside in a crime-ridden inner-city public housing project, where terror and gunshots reigned. She and I never viewed each other as "the other" across a chasm of misunderstanding, because there was a sharing of core values (Solomon, 1983) that became discernible once she and her life were no longer out of control. It would appear that Ms. M and I shared a bicultural perspective: With very few similar life experiences, I emotionally and empathically comprehended her experiences with poverty, racism, domestic violence, victimization, and subjugation as a woman, and she shared my valuation of education for women and their children, hard work, financial self-sufficiency, and (last but not least) insight-oriented psychotherapy. On the strength of her prior course of treatment, she returned to confer with her prior doctor before taking the radical step of surrendering her child to the child welfare system. Nevertheless, despite her appropriate consultation, I was amazed and impressed with Ms. M's commitment to therapy and motivation for help and change for her child and herself. In over 2 years of therapy, except for illness, she never missed or canceled a session for Joy and/or herself, no matter how severe the weather and despite the early hour of 8:00 A.M. for her appointments (to accommodate getting Joy to school and herself to work as early as possible on appointment days). Because of our most positive and productive working relationship and therapeutic alliance, the end phase was stressful.

The time of termination was a period of ambivalent holding on and letting go, on both the mother's and my parts. We both felt and spoke of the real sense of pending loss of a significant real relationship, in which we'd shared a private and most compelling and successful journey. Ms. M believed she had been helped both in her personal treatment, and by me in her child-focused contacts, to find and change her personal identity from a victimized, overwhelmed, abused black wife and mother to that of a black woman "on her way"—acquiring better self-control, parenting skills, and self-knowledge, so that she could make reasoned and gratifying romantic choices. She had also sought and obtained concrete items in her upwardly mobile struggle, and these included education, training, decent housing, and a car. As noted earlier, I often felt intense idealizing countertransferential responses, which I believe included both the mother and her child.

We parted on a most positive note, knowing that I would remain available to Ms. M and to Joy. The mother felt gratified by what she experienced as keen racial sensitivity on my part, and on the part of her individual therapist. We both were perceived as helping to "isolate as well as synthesize the issues of race and gender as markers and organizers for the vicissitudes of [her] being" (Thompson, 1996, p. 138). In addition, Ms. M was gratified that she'd received help and support in regard to acquiring marketable skills, which enabled her to become self-sufficient (Williams, 1990). Indeed, she and I often joked about our shared views that therapy and education are both "passports to freedom."

TERMINATION WITH JOY

During the concluding period of her treatment, Joy and I both experienced a sense of sadness and some degree of anxiety about the pending loss of a special, precious, and private relationship. There was also a sense of pride and pleasure at what had been accomplished, and termination was viewed as a kind of graduation achievement, based on Joy's firmly establishing a progressive line of development (A. Freud, 1962).

Anna Freud later distinguished between the handling of termination for the child and the adult patient:

> It never seemed quire logical to me that terminating a child analysis should involve the complete separation from the analyst that it usually does for adult patients. With children there is the loss of a real object as well as the loss of the transference object, and this complicates matters. To make an absolute break from a certain date onward merely sets up another separation and an unnecessary one. If normal progress is achieved, the child will detach himself anyway, in the course of time, just as children outgrow their nursery school teachers, their school teachers and their friends at certain stages. (A. Freud, quoted in Sandler et al., 1980, p. 243)

Thus she recommended a gradual detachment, with reduction of visits and continual availability of the analyst as a benign background figure.

In child therapy, the focus during termination is less on transference phenomena and more on the here-and-now, real relationship of clinician and child. Thus Joy and I worked out a gradual disengagement, with assurances of my ongoing availability. Although there were episodes of regression and brief reappearances of some symptoms, such as temper eruptions, they were short-lived. Following an early summer termination, Joy expressed wishes to see me again. This was handled via a month of regular weekly appointments in the fall. Her physical growth and apparent emotional growth over the summer were striking, and she had maintained the changes and improvements she had made during her treatment. Her attendance in a summer camp day care program was presented by Joy and her mother as gratifying and positive, with the acquisition of athletic and social skills and more friendships.

In working out the termination, Joy constructed a "book" reviewing her experiences in therapy, which I present below. It demonstrates with vivid clarity how well a very young child understood the reasons she was brought to a therapist; she also poignantly recounted a 61/2-year-old's view of her treatment goals and gains. The "book," when she completed it, touched me greatly. Indeed, I often felt moved almost to tears in the last month or so, at the end of each session when we'd part, and we both knew we had fewer and fewer sessions left.

Joy's Book

Once upon a time a little girl was almost 5 years old. She was not very happy. She would cry and fight with her mommy. She would not sleep alone. She would get mad a lot. Her mommy loved her very much and did not want the fights. She did not want her child to be so sad and mad. She took her little girl to a therapist. The little girl and the therapist worked hard together. They played and talked together for two years. Slowly the little girl became happier. She did not have tantrums, and she and her Mommy did not fight. They were calmer. The little girl got a little older and was more grown up. She could sleep alone and talk about how she felt. She hardly ever yelled, even when she was angry. She learned to read and sing in a choir.

The little girl's name is Joy M. Her mother's name is Pat M. The therapist's name is Ms. M. We all have the initial "M."

Joy cried in therapy sometimes. She also had fun, sang and danced and colored pictures. Now they quit coming to see each other, because everyone got along better. They were happy with each other. All is well.

Epilogue

In recent years, the integration of numerous psychotherapeutic techniques has been emphasized as the emerging trend in the delivery of mental health services. Comas-Díaz (1994) notes that the Society for the Exploration of Psychotherapy Integration established the *Journal of Psychotherapy Integration* in 1991 to increase understanding of the process of change and to improve the effectiveness of psychotherapy. She notes that Okun (1990), among many others, advocates integration and pluralism in psychotherapy; the emphasis is on clinicians' need to find multiple ways to treat clients by selection of methods from different theoretical schools. Comas-Díaz goes on to state that this integrative and comprehensive perspective is particularly essential in providing services for clients of color, in that the integrative approach

> reconciles psycho-therapeutic process variables with the dual [gender and race] and multiple group membership of [clients] of color. . . . The integrative approach acknowledges the confluence of the therapist's and the client's realities. Given that such confluence is associated within the dyadic encounter, the therapeutic relationship is presented

237

as an illustration of the integration of essential process variables into a
gender-, ethnicity-, and race-informed clinical work. (p. 287)

In other words, integration combines traditional psychotherapeutic models with sociocultural, ethnic, racial, and gender contexts. The reality of belonging to more than one disenfranchised
group (e.g., being a woman and an ethnic minority) is a paramount
consideration within the integrative approach. Consequently, such
clients' experiences of racism, sexism, identity conflicts, oppression,
migration/acculturation, environmental stressors, and internalized
colonization have become important considerations in the delivery
of appropriate clinical services (Comas-Díaz, 1994).

I have utilized a psychoanalytic/psychodynamic approach, with
particular reliance on more recent theories—namely, self psychology
and theories of intersubjectivity—as the primary basis of my assessments and interventions. However, I have not ignored older paradigms such as drive theory and ego psychology, especially in the assessment of some of the cases presented in this book. Furthermore, a
flexible and pluralistic approach encourages the integrative use of
feminist and empowerment theory, a strength perspective, family
theory, narrative theory, and Falicov's (1998) multidimensional eco-
systemic comparative approach (which is based on the above-
described concept that each person's cultural identity consists of
multiple forms of belonging and participation and identification, including race, ethnicity, gender, religion, occupation, and socioeconomic status). Other perspectives utilized in cross-cultural treatment are not based on psychology or psychoanalysis, but come from
sociology, anthropology, and linguistics, as described in Chapter 2.

The therapeutic relationship has been identified as the critical
variable in working with people of color. For me, the most helpful
bridges over differences in the cross-cultural therapeutic dyad are
empathy and awareness of the reciprocal interplay between two or
more subjective worlds. Thus I have come to find intersubjectivity
theory and self psychology (both relational theories) essential in
cross-cultural work, since both are reliant on empathy and introspection as crucial guiding principles.

As noted throughout this book, empathy includes both affective and cognitive components. The affective component involves feelings of emotional connectedness to the client and a capacity to take in and contain the feelings of the client (Kaplan, 1991), "which is similar to a subjective and phenomenological experience of being like the client" (Comas-Díaz, 1994, p. 294). The cognitive component involves an intellectual understanding of the client, as captured in Kleinman's (1989) concept of "empathic witnessing": The therapist in an unmatched dyad recognizes his or her ethnic/cultural ignorance of the client's reality, and reaffirms, through such witnessing, the client's experience and reality. At times it can be difficult to be empathic with those who are culturally different, and this must be recognized via introspection and self-awareness in the management of the therapeutic relationship.

In a passage I have quoted in full in Chapter 5, Kohut, the father of self psychology, defined "empathy" as "the recognition of the self in the other, . . . the expansion of the self to include the other, . . . and the accepting, confirming and understanding human echo evoked by the self" (cited in Ornstein, 1978, p. 84). According to Stolorow (1994), the intersubjective field is broader and more inclusive than the self–selfobject relationship of self psychology; it is a more broad-based striving to organize and order experiences. As I have noted in Chapter 2, the intersubjectivity theorists conclude that the transference and countertransference constitute a reciprocal, mutually influential system (Stolorow, Brandchaft, Atwood, & Lachmann, 1987). Within this two-person paradigm, the clinician's role in the intersubjective exchange is acknowledged. Thus an addition to the concept of empathy is the intersubjectivity theorists' recognition of the contributing role of the therapist's own biases, action, inactions, and psychology. I agree with Perez Foster (1996) and Altman (1996) that this recognition is essential in the treatment of any patient whose class, religion, culture, race, and/or value system differs from that of the therapist.

Just as important as the recognition of differences between patient and therapist is the appreciation of sameness between groups. Montabo (1994) notes that therapeutic relatedness requires the perception of kinship, which is the heart of our common humanity. This text attempts to demonstrate the appreciation of both diversity and sameness between client and clinician. I can only hope that I have achieved my goal—namely, the presentation of connectedness in the professional relationship and the underlying core of humanity between me and my patients, who have taught me about their respective cultures. I increasingly consider ethnic/cultural/racial influences as central and necessary to the theory and practice of psychotherapy, and as of equal importance to models focusing on intrapsychic and interpersonal variables. I have attempted to offer portraits that individualize my patients, to avoid any sort of stereotyping or homogeneous view of any ethnic or racial group. While familiar with characteristics of particular cultures, I have attempted to demonstrate a stance of "not-knowing" and curiosity. This has stimulated my efforts to engage in a dialogue with my patients that resembles Falicov's (1998) concept of the "double discourse," "an ability to see the univeral similarities that unite us beyond color, class, ethnicity, and gender while simultaneously recognizing and respecting culture-specific differences that exist due to color, class, ethnicity and gender" (p. 275).

I appreciate having had the opportunity to work with and learn from my patients, and to have been given permission by several to present our private and special journey together. (The remaining cases, as noted in the Preface, are disguised amalgams of persons and situations drawn from decades of cross-cultural psychotherapy.) I have attempted to offer accessible tools and concepts for seasoned clinicians as well as novices, by emphasizing theoretical evolution and clinical applications that I hope will give my readers new insights into cross-cultural psychotherapy. It is my hope that this text has allowed the process of such treatment and the life experiences of my patients to come alive, in order to augment my readers' clinical practice experience, whether or not there is total agreement on the treatment methods and assessments presented.

References

Abell, N., & McDonnell, J. C. (1990). Preparing for practice: Motivations, expectations and aspirations of the MSW class of 1990. *Journal of Social Work Education, 26,* 57–64.

Abramovitz, S. I., & Murray, J. (1983). Race effects in psychotherapy. In J. Murray & P. Abramson (Eds.), *Bias in psychotherapy* (pp. 215–255). New York: Praeger.

Adams, P. L. (1970). Dealing with racism in biracial psychiatry. *Journal of the American Academy of Child Psychiatry, 9,* 33–43.

Alexander, F. (1963). The dynamics of psychotherapy in the light of learning theory. *American Journal of Psychiatry, 120,* 440–448.

Altman, N. (1995). *The analyst in the inner city: Race, class and culture through a psychoanalytic lens.* Hillsdale, NJ: Analytic Press.

Altman, N. (1996). The accommodation of diversity in psychoanalysis. In R. Perez Foster, M. Moskowitz, & R. A. Javier (Eds.), *Reaching across boundaries of culture and class: Widening the scope of psychotherapy* (pp. 196–224). Northvale, NJ: Jason Aronson.

American Psychiatric Association. (1994). *Diagnostic and statistical manual of mental disorders* (4th ed.). Washington, DC: Author.

Anderson, C. M., & Stewart, S. (1983). *Mastering resistance: A practical guide to family therapy.* New York: Guilford Press.

Anderson, H., & Goolishian, H. A. (1988). Human systems in linguistic systems: Preliminary and evolving ideas about the implications for clinical theory. *Family Process, 27,* 371–393.

241

Anderson, H., & Goolishian, H. A. (1992). The client is the expert: A not-knowing approach to therapy. In S. McNamee & K. Gergen (Eds.), *Therapy as social construction* (pp. 25–39). Newbury Park, CA: Sage.

Anderson, L. P. (1991). Acculturative stress: A theory of relevance to black Americans. *Clinical Psychology Review, 11*, 685–702.

Aron, L. (1996). *A meeting of minds.* Hillsdale, NJ: Analytic Press.

Atkinson, D. R. (1985). A meta-review of research on cross-cultural counseling and psychotherapy. *Journal of Multi-Cultural Counseling and Development, 1*, 138–153.

Atkinson, D. R., Morten, G., & Sue, D. W. (Eds.). (1979). *Counseling American minorities: A cross-cultural perspective.* Dubuque, IA: William C. Brown.

Atkinson, D. R., Morten, G., & Sue, D. W. (1998). *Counseling American minorities* (5th ed.). Boston: McGraw-Hill.

Atwood, G., & Stolorow, R. D. (1984). *Structures of subjectivity: Explorations in psychoanalytic phenomenology.* Hillsdale, NJ: Analytic Press.

Bacal, H. A. (1979). *Empathic lag in the analyst and its relation to negative therapeutic reaction.* Paper presented at the 31st International Psychoanalytic Congress, New York.

Bacal, H. A. (1985). Optimal responsiveness and the therapeutic process. In H. A. Goldberg (Ed.), *Progress in self psychology* (Vol. 1, pp. 202–227). New York: Guilford Press.

Bacal, H. A. (1990). Heinz Kohut. In H. A. Bacal & K. M. Newman (Eds.), *Theories of object relations: Bridges to self psychology* (pp. 221–273). New York: Columbia University Press.

Bacal, H. A. (Ed.). (1998a). *Optimal responsiveness: How therapists heal their patients.* Northvale, NJ: Jason Aronson.

Bacal, H. A. (1998b). Optimal responsiveness and the specificity of self object experience. In H. A. Bacal (Ed.), *Optimal responsiveness: How therapists heal their patients* (pp. 141–170). Northvale, NJ: Jason Aronson.

Balint, M. (1968). *The basic fault.* London: Tavistock.

Barth, D. (1991). When the patient abuses food. In H. Jackson (Ed.), *Using self psychology in psychotherapy* (pp. 223–242). Northvale, NJ: Jason Aronson.

Basch, M. (1980). *Doing psychotherapy.* New York: Basic Books.

Basch, M. (1986). How does analysis cure?: An appreciation. *Psychoanalytic Inquiry, 6*, 403–428.

Beasley, L. (1972). A beginning attempt to eradicate racist attitudes. *Social Casework, 53*, 9–13.

Beebe, B., & Lachmann, F. (1988a). The contribution of the mother–infant mutual influence to the origins of self and object representations. *Psychoanalytic Psychology, 5*, 305–337.

Beebe, B., & Lachmann, F. (1988b). Mother–infant mutual influence and precursors of psychic structure. In A. Goldberg (Ed.), *Frontiers in self psychology* (pp. 3–25). Hillsdale, NJ: Analytic Press.

Bell, D., & Evan, S. (1981). *Counseling the black client* (Professional Education, No. 5). Minneapolis, MN: Hazelden Foundation.

Bell, E. (1990). The bicultural life experience of career oriented black women. *Journal of Organizational Behavior, 4,* 459–477.

Beren, P. (1998). Narcissistic disorders in children. In P. Beren (Ed.), *Narcissistic disorders in children and adolescents: Diagnosis and treatment* (pp. 151–165). Northvale, NJ: Jason Aronson.

Bernard, V. W. (1953). Psychoanalysis and members of minority groups. *Journal of the American Psychoanalytic Association, 1,* 256–267.

Bernfeld, S. (1928). *Sisyphos, ader veber die grenzen de erziehung.* Vienna: Internationale Verinig ung fuer Psychoanalysis.

Berzoff, J., Flanagan, L. M., & Hertz, P. (1996). *Inside out and outside in: Psychodynamic clinical theory and practice.* Northvale, NJ: Jason Aronson.

Bettelheim, B. (1983). *Freud and man's soul.* New York: Knopf.

Billingsley, A., & Giovannoni, J. (1972). *Children of the storm: Black children and the American child welfare system.* New York: Harcourt Brace Jovanovich.

Bion, W. R. (1955). Language of the schizophrenic. In M. Klein, P. Heimann, & R. E. Money-Kyrle (Eds.), *New directions in psychoanalysis* (pp. 230–239). London: Tavistock.

Blanck, G., & Blanck, R. (1979a). *Ego psychology I: Theory and practice.* New York: Columbia University Press.

Blanck, G., & Blanck, R. (1979b). *Ego psychology II: Psychoanalytic developmental psychology.* New York: Columbia University Press.

Blauner, R. (1992). Talking past each other: Black and white language of race. *American Prospect, 10,* 55–64.

Blos, P. (1962). *On adolescence.* New York: Free Press.

Blos, P. (1972). The epigenesis of the adult neurosis. *Psychoanalytic Study of the Child, 27,* 106–135.

Blos, P. (1983). The contribution of psychoanalysis to the psychotherapy of adolescence. In M. Sugar (Ed.), *Adolescent psychiatry: Vol. 11. Developmental and clinical studies* (pp. 104–124). Chicago: University of Chicago Press.

Boyd-Franklin, N. (1989). *Black families in therapy: A multisystems approach.* New York: Guilford Press.

Boyd-Franklin, N. (1991). Recurrent themes in treatment of African-American women in group therapy. *Women and Therapy, 11*(2), 25–40.

Brandchaft, B. (1983). The negativism of the negative therapeutic reaction and the psychology of the self. In A. Goldberg (Ed.), *The future of psychoanalysis* (pp. 327–359). New York: International Universities Press.

Butler, A. C. (1992). The attractions of private practice. *Journal of Social Work Education, 28,* 47–60.

Buxbaum, E. (1950). Technique of terminating analysis. *International Journal of Psycho-Analysis, 31,* 184–190.

Calnek, M. (1970). Racial factors in the countertransference: The black therapist and the black client. *American Journal of Orthopsychiatry, 40,* 39–46.

Campbell, R. (1981). *Psychiatric dictionary* (5th ed.). New York: Oxford University Press.

Cangelosi, D. (1997). *Saying goodbye in child psychotherapy: Planned, unplanned and premature endings.* Northvale, NJ: Jason Aronson.

Canino, I. (1990). *Working with people from Hispanic backgrounds.* Paper presented at the Cross-Cultural Psychotherapy Conference, Hahnemann University, Philadelphia.

Carkhuff, R. R., & Pierce, R. (1967). The differential effects of therapists' race and class upon patient depth of self-exploration in the initial clinical interview. *Journal of Consulting Psychology, 31,* 632–634.

Casement, P. C. (1990). *Learning from the patient.* New York: Guilford Press.

Chestang, L. (1979). Competencies and knowledge in clinical social work: A dual perspective. In P. L. Ewalt (Ed.), *Toward a definition of clinical social work* (pp. 1–12). Washington, DC: National Association of Social Workers.

Children's Defense Fund. (1985). *Black and white children in America: Key facts.* Washington, DC: Author.

Chin, J. L. (1988). Institutional racism and mental health: An Asian-American perspective. In O. A. Barbarin, P. R. Good, C. M. Pharr, & J. A. Siskind (Eds.), *Institutional racism and community competence* (pp. 44–55). Washington, DC: U.S. Government Printing Office.

Chin, J. L. (1994). Psychodynamic approaches. In L. Comas-Díaz & B. Greene (Eds.), *Women of color: Integrating ethnic and gender identities in psychotherapy* (pp. 194–222). New York: Guilford Press.

Clark, K. B., & Clark, M. K. (1947). Racial identification and preferences in Negro children. In T. M. Newcomb & E. L. Hostley (Eds.), *Readings in social psychology* (pp. 168–178). New York: Holt, Rinehart & Winston.

Cohan, D. (1998). *Towards an understanding of the sociology of race.* Unpublished manuscript.

Coleman, D. (2000). The therapeutic alliance in multi-cultural practice. *Psychoanalytic Social Work, 7*(2), 65–91.

Comas-Díaz, L. (1987). Ethnocultural identification in psychotherapy. *Psychiatry, 50,* 232–241.

Comas-Díaz, L. (1988). Cross-cultural mental health treatment. In L. Comas-Díaz & E. H. Griffith (Eds.), *Clinical guidelines in cross-cultural mental health* (pp. 335–362). New York: Wiley.

Comas-Díaz, L. (1994). An integrative approach. In L. Comas-Díaz & B. Greene (Eds.), *Women of color: Integrating ethnic and gender identity in psychotherapy* (pp. 287–318). New York: Guilford Press.

Comas-Díaz, L., & Greene, B. (1994a). Overview: An ethnocultural mosaic. In L. Comas-Díaz & B. Greene (Eds.), *Women of color: Integrating ethnic and gender identities in psychotherapy* (pp. 3–9). New York: Guilford Press.

Comas-Díaz, L., & Greene, B. (1994b). Women of color with professional status. In L. Comas-Díaz & B. Greene (Eds.), *Women of color: Integrating ethnic and gender identity in psychotherapy* (pp. 347–388). New York: Guilford Press.

Comas-Díaz, L., & Jacobsen, F. M. (1991). Ethnocultural transference and countertransference in the therapeutic dyad. *American Journal of Orthopsychiatry, 61*(3), 392–402.

Comas-Díaz, L., & Minrath, M. (1985). Psychotherapy with ethnic minority borderline clients. *Psychotherapy, 22*(2), 418–426.

Cooper, A. M., Frances, A. J., & Sacks, M. H. (1986). The psychoanalytic model. In A. M. Cooper, A. J. Frances, & M. H. Sacks (Eds.), *Psychiatry: Vol. 1. The personality disorders and neurosis* (pp. 1–16). New York: Basic Books.

Cooper, M., & Lesser, J. (1997). How race affects the helping process: A case of cross-racial therapy. *Clinical Social Work Journal, 25*(3), 323–335.

Cox, D. (1985). Welfare services for migrants: Can they be better planned? *International Migration Review, 23*(1), 73–93.

Cross, T. L., Bazron, B. J., Dennis, K. W., & Isaacs, M. R. (1989). *Towards a culturally competent system of care.* Washington, DC: CASSPT Technical Assistance Center.

Curtis, H. (1980). The concept of therapeutic alliance: Implications for the widening scope. In H. Blum (Ed.), *Psychoanalytic exploration of technique: Discourse on the theory and therapy* (pp. 159–192). New York: International Universities Press. (Original work published 1977)

Davanloo, H. (Ed.). (1980). *Short-term dynamic psychotherapy.* Northvale, NJ: Jason Aronson.

Davidson, J. R. (1992). Theories about black–white interracial marriage: A clinical perspective. *Journal of Multi-Cultural Counseling and Development, 20*(4), 150–157.

Davis, L., & Procter, E. K. (1989). *Race, gender and class: Guidelines for practice with individuals, families and groups.* Englewood Cliffs, NJ: Prentice-Hall.

Dean, R. G. (2000). The myth of cross-cultural competence: A clinical vignette. In *Proceedings of the International Social Work Conference, Barcelona, Spain, May 12–15, 2000* (pp. 136–142). New York: Shirley M. Ehrenkranz School of Social Work, New York University.

Deitz, J. (1991). When the patient is depressed. In H. Jackson (Ed.), *Using self psychology in psychotherapy* (pp. 193–201). Northvale, NJ: Jason Aronson.

DeLaCancela, V. (1985). Towards a sociocultural psychotherapy for low income ethnic minorities. *Psychotherapy, 22*(2), 427–435.

Devore, W., & Schlesinger, E. G. (1987). *Ethnic-sensitive social work practice* (2nd ed.). Columbus, OH: Merrill.

Devore, W., & Schlesinger, E. G. (1991). *Ethnic-sensitive social work practice.* New York: Macmillan.

Devore, W., & Schlesinger, E. G. (1999). *Ethnic-sensitive social work practice* (5th ed.). Boston: Allyn & Bacon.

DeWald, P. (1967). The termination of psychotherapy. *Psychiatry Digest, 38,* 33–46.

Drachman, D. (1982). A stage of migration framework as applied to recent joint émigrés. *Journal of Multicultural Social Work, 2*(1), 63–78.

Drachman, D., & Ryan, A. S. (1991). Immigrants and refugees. In A. Gitterman (Ed.), *Handbook of social work practice with vulnerable populations* (pp. 618–646). New York: Columbia University Press.

Edward, J. (1996). Listening, hearing and understanding in psychoanalytically oriented treatment. In J. Edward & J. Sanville (Eds.), *Fostering healing and growth: A psychoanalytic social work approach* (pp. 23–45). Northvale, NJ: Jason Aronson.

Eissler, R., Freud, A., Kris, M., & Solnit, A. (Eds.). (1977). *An anthology of the psychoanalytic study of the child: Psychoanalytic assessment—A diagnostic profile*. New Haven, CT: Yale University Press.

Elbow, M. (1987). The memory book: Facilitating termination with children. *Social Casework, 68,* 180–183.

Elson, M. (1984). Parenthood and the transformation of narcissism in parenthood. In R. Cohen, B. Cohler, & S. Weissman (Eds.), *Parenthood: A psychodynamic perspective* (pp. 297–314). New York: Guilford Press.

Elson, M. (1986). *Self psychology in clinical social work.* New York: Norton.

Espin, O. (1994). Feminist approaches. In L. Comas-Díaz & B. Greene (Eds.), *Women of color: Integrating ethnic and gender identity in psychotherapy* (pp. 265–286). New York: Guilford Press.

Falicov, C. J. (Ed.). (1983). *Cultural perspectives in family therapy.* Rockville, MD: Aspen.

Falicov, C. J. (1998). *Latino families in therapy: A guide to multicultural practice.* New York: Guilford Press.

Ferenczi, S. (1955). The problem of the termination of the analysis. In M. Balint (Ed.), *Final contributions to the problems and methods of psychoanalysis* (pp. 77–87). New York: Basic Books. (Original work published 1927)

Firestone, S. (1974). Termination of psychoanalysis of adults: A review of the literature. *Journal of the American Psychoanalytic Association, 20,* 873–894.

Firestone, S. (1978). *Termination in psychoanalysis.* New York: International Universities Press.

Fischer, N. (1971). An interracial analysis: Transference and countertransference significance. *Journal of the American Psychoanalytic Association, 19,* 736–745.

Fish, J. (1996). *Culture and therapy: An integrated approach.* Northvale, NJ: Jason Aronson.

Fortune, A. E., Pearlingo, B., & Rochelle, C. D. (1992). Reactions to termination of individual treatment. *Social Work, 37*(2), 171–178.

Freeman, E. M. (1990a). The black families' life cycle: Operationalizing a strength perspective. In S. L. Logan, E. M. Freeman, & R. G. McRoy (Eds.), *Social work practice with black families* (pp. 55–72). New York: Longman.

Freeman, E. M. (1990b). Theoretical perspectives for practice with black families. In S. M. L. Logan, E. M. Freeman, & R. G. McRoy (Eds.), *Social work practice with black families* (pp. 38–52). New York: Longman.

Freud, A. (1946). *The ego and the mechanisms of defense.* New York: International Universities Press.

Freud, A. (1951). *The psychoanalytic treatment of children* (3rd ed.; N. Proctor, Trans.). London: Anglo Books.

Freud, A. (1962). Assessment of childhood disturbances. *Psychoanalytic Study of the Child, 17,* 149–158.

Freud, A. (1965). *The writings of Anna Freud VI: Normality and pathology in childhood—Assessments of development.* New York: International Universities Press.

Freud, A. (1971). The infantile neurosis: Genetic and dynamic considerations. In *The psychoanalytic study of the child* (p. 26). New York: Quadrangle Press.

Freud, A. (1977). The symptomatology of childhood: A preliminary classification. In R. Eissler, A. Freud, M. Kris, & A. Solnit (Eds.), *An anthology of the psychoanalytic study of the child: Psychoanalytic assessment—A diagnostic profile* (pp. 31–53). New Haven, CT: Yale University Press.

Freud, A., Nagera, H., & Freud, W. E. (1965). Metapsychological assessment of the adult personality: The adult profile. In R. S. Eissler, A. Freud, M. Kris, & A. V. Solnit (Eds.), *An anthology of the psychoanalytic study of the child: Psychoanalytic assessment—A diagnostic profile* (pp. 82–114). New Haven, CT: Yale University Press.

Freud, S. (1926). Inhibitions, symptoms, and anxiety. In J. Strachey (Ed. & Trans.), *Standard edition of the complete psychological works of Sigmund Freud* (Vol. 20, pp. 87–151). London: Hogarth Press.

Freud, S. (1937). Analysis terminable and interminable. In S. Freud, *Collected papers* (Vol. 5, pp. 316–357). London: Hogarth Press.

Freud, S. (1952). *A general introduction to psychoanalysis.* New York: Washington Square Press. (Original work published 1900)

Freud, S. (1958). The dynamics of transference. In J. Strachey (Ed. & Trans.), *The standard edition of the complete works of Sigmund Freud* (Vol. 12, pp. 97–108). London: Hogarth Press. (Original work published 1912)

Freud, S. (1958). Observations on transference love. In J. Strachey (Ed. & Trans.), *The standard edition of the complete works of Sigmund Freud* (Vol. 12, pp. 157–171). London: Hogarth Press. (Original work published 1915)

Furman, E. (1980). Transference and externalization in latency. *Psychoanalytic Study of the Child, 35,* 267–284.

Garcia, R. (1979). The need for culturally relevant training and materials. *Journal of Hispanic Issues, 9,* 10–36.

Gardner, G. (1990). *Working with persons from African-American backgrounds.* Paper presented at the Cross-Cultural Psychotherapy Conference, Hahnemann University, Philadelphia.

Garland, J. A. Jones, H. E., & Kolodny, R. L. (1973). A model for stages of development in social work groups. In S. Bernstein (Ed.), *Explorations in group work: Essays in theory and practice* (pp. 17–71). Boston: Milford House.

Garrett, A. (1972). *Interviewing* (2nd ed.). New York: Family Service America.

Gates, H. (1994). The use of anti-Semitism. In P. Berman (Ed.), *Blacks and Jews: Alliances and arguments* (pp. 217–228). New York: Delacorte.

Germain, C. B., & Gitterman, A. (1980). *The life model of social work practice.* New York: Columbia University Press.

Gill, M. (1982). *Analysis of transference* (Vol. 1). New York: International Universities Press.

Giovacchini, P. (1985). Countertransference and the severely disturbed adolescent. In M. Sugar, S. Feinstein, J. Loony, A. Schwartzberg, & A. Sorosky (Eds.), *Adolescent psychiatry Vol. 12: Developmental and clinical studies* (pp. 447–448). Chicago: University of Chicago Press.

Glenn, M. (1971). Separation anxiety: When the therapist leaves the patient. *American Journal of Psychotherapy, 25,* 437–445.

Goldberg, E. L., Myers, W. A., & Zeifman, I. (1974). Some observations on three interracial analyses. *International Journal of Psycho-Analysis, 55,* 495–500.

Goldstein, E. G., & Noonan, M. (1999). *Short-term treatment and social work practice: An integrative perspective.* New York: Free Press.

Goleman, D. (1995, December 5). Making room on the couch for culture. *The New York Times,* p. C-6.

Gordon, M. M. (1988). *The scope of sociology.* New York: Oxford University Press.

Gould, R. (1978). Students' experience with the termination phase of individual treatment. *Smith College Studies in Social Work, 48*(3), 235–269.

Grayson, H. (1970). Grief reaction to the relinquishing of unfulfilled wishes. *American Journal of Psychotherapy, 24,* 287–295.

Green, R.-J. (1998). Race and the field of family therapy. In M. McGoldrick (Ed.), *Re-visioning family therapy* (pp. 93–110). New York: Guilford Press.

Greenson, R. R. (1965). The working alliance and the transference neurosis. *Psychoanalytic Quarterly, 34,* 155–181.

Griffin, M. S. (1977). The influence of race on the psychotherapeutic relationship. *Psychiatry, 40,* 27–40.

Guntrip, H. (1975). My experience of analysis with Fairbairn and Winnicott. *International Review of Psychoanalysis, 2,* 145–156.

Gutheil, I. (1993). Rituals and termination procedures. *Smith College Studies in Social Work, 63*(2), 163–175.

Gutierrez, L. M. (1990). Working with women of color: An empowerment perspective. *Social Work, 37*(8), 149–153.

Hacker, A. (1994). Jewish racism, black anti-Semitism. In P. Berman (Ed.), *Blacks and Jews: Alliances and arguments* (pp. 154–163). New York: Delacorte Press.

Hamilton, J. A. (1989). Emotional consequences of victimization and discrimination in "special populations" of women. In P. Parry (Ed.), *Women's disorders* (pp. 35–53). Philadelphia: W. B. Saunders.

Hamilton, J. A., & Jensuold, M. (1992). Personality, psychopathology and depression in women. In L. S. Brown & M. Ballou (Eds.), *Personality and psychopathology: Feminist reappraisals* (pp. 116–143). New York: Guilford Press.

Hanna, E. A. (1998). The role of the therapist's subjectivity: Using countertransference in psychotherapy. *Journal of Analytic Social Work, 5*(4), 1–24.

Hepworth, D. H., & Larson, A. (1986). *Direct social work practice: Theory and skills* (2nd ed.). Chicago: Dorsey Press.

Herman, J. L. (1992). *Trauma and recovery.* New York: Basic Books.

Ho, M. K., & McDowell, E. (1973). The black worker, white client relationship. *Clinical Social Work Journal, 1,* 161–167.

Hoffman, I. (1996). The intimate and ironic authority of the psychoanalytic presence. *Psychoanalytic Quarterly, 65,* 102–136.

Hollingshead, H. B., & Redlich, F. C. (1958). *Social class and mental illness.* New York: Wiley.

hooks, b. (1989). *Talking back: Thinking feminist, thinking black.* Boston: South End Press.

Ivey, A. E., Ivey, M. B., & Simek-Morgan, I. (1993). *Counseling and psychotherapy: A multi-cultural perspective* (3rd ed.). Needham Heights, MA: Allyn & Bacon.

Jackson, A. M. (1983). Treatment issues for black patients. *Psychotherapy: Theory, Research and Practice, 20,* 143–151.

Jackson, L. C. (1999). Ethnocultural resistance to multi-cultural training: Students and faculty. *Cultural Diversity and Ethnic Minority Psychology, 5*(1), 27–36.

Javier, R. A. (1990). The suitability of insight oriented therapy for the Hispanic poor. *American Journal of Psychoanalysis, 50,* 305–318.

Javier, R. A. (1996). Psychodynamic treatment with the urban poor. In R. Perez Foster, M. Moskowitz, & R. A. Javier (Eds.), *Reaching across boundaries of culture and class: Widening the scope of psychotherapy* (pp. 93–113). Northvale, NJ: Jason Aronson.

Jenkins, A. H. (1990). Dynamics of the relationship in clinical work with African-American clients. *Group, 14*(1), 36–43.

Jones, A. C. (1985). Psychological functioning in Black Americans: A conceptual guide for all in psychotherapy. *Psychotherapy, 22,* 363–369.

Jones, E. E. (1985). Psychotherapy and counseling with black clients. In Pedersen (Ed.), *Handbook of cross-cultural counseling and therapy* (pp. 173–179). Westport, CT: Greenwood Press.

Jordan, J. V. (1991). Empathy and self-boundaries. In J. V. Jordan, A. G. Kaplan, J. B. Miller, I. P. Stiver, & J. L. Surrey (Eds.), *Women's growth in connection: Writings from the Stone Center* (pp. 67–80). New York: Guilford Press.

Kadushin, A. (1972). The racial factor in the interview. *Social Work, 17,* 88–98.

Kanuha, V. (1994). Women of color in battering relationships. In L. Comas-Díaz & B. Greene (Eds.), *Women of color: Integrating ethnic and gender identities in psychotherapy* (pp. 428–454). New York: Guilford Press.

Kaplan, A. G. (1991). Female or male therapists for women: New formulations. In J. V. Jordan, A. G. Kaplan, J. B. Miller, I. P. Stiver, & J. L. Surrey (Eds.), *Women's growth in connection: Writings from the Stone Center* (pp. 268–282). New York: Guilford Press.

Kautz, E. (1976). Can agencies train for racial awareness? *Child Welfare, 55,* 547–551.

Keller, S. (1975). *Uprooting and social change: The role of refugees in development.* Delhi, India: Manohar Book Service.

Kessler, J. (1966). *Psychopathology of childhood.* Englewood Cliffs, NJ: Prentice-Hall.

Kleinman, A. (1989, May 19). *Culture, suffering and psychotherapy.* Paper presented at the Psychotherapy of Diversity: Cross-Cultural Treatment Issues conference, Boston.

Kohrman, R. (1969). Panel report on "Problems of termination in child analysis": Annual meeting of the American Psychoanalytic Association. Boston, MA: May 10, 1968. *Journal of the American Psychoanalytic Association, 28,* 191–205.

Kohut, H. (1959). Introspection, empathy and psychoanalysis. *Journal of the American Psychoanalytic Association, 7,* 459–483.

Kohut, H. (1971). *The analysis of the self; a systematic approach to the psychoanalytic treatment of narcissistic personality disorders.* New York: International Universities Press.

Kohut, H. (1977). *The restoration of the self.* New York: International Universities Press.

Kohut, H. (1978). *The search for the self: Selected writings of Heinz Kohut, 1950–1978* (Vol. 1; P. Ornstein, Ed.). New York: International Universities Press.

Kohut, H. (1982). Introspection, empathy and the semi-circle of mental health. *International Journal of Psycho-Analysis, 63,* 395–407.

Kohut, H. (1984). *How does analysis cure?* (A. Goldberg & P. Stepansky, Eds.). Chicago: University of Chicago Press.

Kohut, H., & Wolf, E. S. (1978). Disorders of the self and their treatment. *International Journal of Psycho-analysis, 57,* 413–425.

Kris, E. (1956). On some vicissitudes of insight in psychoanalysis. *International Journal of Psychoanalysis, 37,* 445–455.

LaFromboise, T., Coleman, H. L. K., & Gerton, J. (1993). Psychological impact and biculturalism: Evidence and theory. *Psychological Bulletin, 114*(3), 395–412.

Laird, J. (1998). Theorizing culture: Narrative ideas and practice principles. In M. McGoldrick (Ed.), *Re-visioning family therapy* (pp. 20–36). New York: Guilford Press.

Langman, P. E. (1999). *Jewish issues in multiculturalism: A handbook for educators and clinicians.* Northvale, NJ: Jason Aronson.

Lazar, S. G. (1998). Optimal responsiveness and enactments. In H.A. Bacall (Ed.), *Optimal responsiveness: How therapists heal their patients* (pp. 213–233). Northvale, NJ: Jason Aronson.

Lerner, M. (1992). *The socialism of fools: Anti-Semitism on the left.* Oakland, CA: Tikkun Books.

Lester, J. (1994). The lives people live. In P. Berman (Ed.), *Blacks and Jews: Alliances and arguments* (pp. 164–177). New York: Delacorte Press.

Levin, D. (1998). Unplanned termination: Pain and consequences. *Journal of Analytic Social Work, 5*(2), 35–46.

Lichtenberg, J. (1983). *Psychoanalysis and infant research.* Hillsdale, NJ: Analytic Press.

Loewald, H. (1962). Internalization, separation, mourning and the superego. *Psychoanalytic Quarterly, 31,* 483–504.

Lu, F. G., Lim, R. F., & Mezzich, J. E. (1995). Issues in the assessment and diagnosis of culturally diverse individuals. In J. Cham & M. Riba (Eds.), *American Psychiatric Press review of psychiatry* (Vol. 14, pp. 477–510). Washington, DC: American Psychiatric Press.

Lum, D. (2000). *Social work practice and people of color: A process stage approach* (4th ed.). Pacific Grove, CA: Brooks/Cole.

Lynch, V. J. (1991). Basic concepts. In H. Jackson (Ed.), *Using self psychology in psychotherapy* (pp. 15–25). Northvale, NJ: Jason Aronson.

Malan, D. H. (1980). The most important development in psychotherapy since the discovery of the unconscious. In H. Davanloo (Ed.), *Short-term dynamic psychotherapy* (pp. 13–24). Northvale, NJ: Jason Aronson.

Maluccio, A , & Marlow, W. (1974). The case for the contract. *Social Work, 19*, 28–35.

Mann, J. (1973). *Time-limited psychotherapy.* Cambridge, MA: Harvard University Press.

Manoleas, P. (1996). Culture and case management. In P. Manoleas (Ed.), *The cross-cultural practice of clinical case management in mental health* (pp. 1–40). Binghamton, NY: Haworth Press.

Marcos, L. R., & Urcuyo, L. (1979). Dynamic psychotherapy with the bilingual patient. *American Journal of Psychotherapy, 33*, 331–338.

Marcus, I. (1980). Countertransference and the psychoanalytic process in children and adolescents. *Psychoanalytic Study of the Child, 35*, 285–298.

Marger, M. N. (1997). *Race and ethnic relations* (4th ed.). Belmont, CA: Wadsworth.

Marmor, J. (1982). Changes in psychoanalytic treatment. In S. Slip (Ed.), *Curative factors in dynamic psychotherapy* (pp. 60–70). New York: McGraw-Hill.

Martin, E. S., & Schurtman, R. (1985). Termination anxiety as it affects the therapist. *Psychotherapy: Theory, Research and Practice, 22*, 92–96.

Mays, V. (1985). The black American and psychotherapy: The dilemma. *Psychotherapy, 22*, 379–387.

McAdoo, H. P. (1981). Patterns of upward mobility in black families. In H. P. McAdoo (Eds.), *Black families* (pp. 155–169). Beverly Hills, CA: Sage.

McCall, M. M., & Wittner, J. (1990). The good news about life history. In H. S. Becker & M. M. McCall (Eds.), *Symbolic interaction and cultural studies* (pp. 46–89). Chicago: University of Chicago Press.

McGill, D. W. (1992). The cultural story in multi-cultural family therapy. *Families in Society, 73*, 339–349.

McGoldrick, M., Pearce, J. K., & Giordano, J. (Eds.). (1982). *Ethnicity and family therapy.* New York: Guilford Press.

McGrath, E., Keita, G. P., Strickland, B. R., & Russo, N. F. (Eds.). (1990). *Women and depression: Risk factors and treatment issues.* Washington, DC: American Psychological Association.

McRoy, R. G., Freeman, E. D., Logan, S. L., & Blackman, B. (1986). Cross-cultural field supervision: Implications for social work education. *Journal of Social Work Education, 22*(1), 50–56.

Meeks, J. (1971). *The fragile alliance: An orientation to the outpatient psychotherapy of the adolescent.* Baltimore: Williams & Wilkins.

Meers, D. (1970). Contributions of a ghetto culture to symptom formation: Psychoanalytic studies of ego anomalies in childhood. *Psychoanalytic Study of the Child, 25,* 209–230.

Meissner, W. W. (1985). Adolescent paranoia: Transference and countertransference issues. *Adolescent Psychiatry, 12,* 478–508.

Messer, S. B., & Warren, C. S. (1995). *Models of brief psychodynamic therapy: A comparative approach.* New York: Guilford Press.

Meyer, C. H. (1993). *Assessment in social work practice.* New York: Columbia University Press.

Middleman, R., & Goldberg, G. (1974). *Social service delivery: A structural approach to practice.* New York: Columbia University Press.

Miliora, M. T. (2000). Beyond empathic failures: Cultural racism and narcissistic trauma and disenfranchisement of grandiosity. *Clinical Social Work Journal, 28*(1), 43–54.

Mishne, J. (1982). The missing system in social work's application of systems theory. *Social Casework, 63*(9), 547–553.

Mishne, J. (1983). *Clinical work with children.* New York: Free Press.

Mishne, J. (1986). *Clinical work with adolescents.* New York: Free Press.

Mishne, J. (1989). Individual treatment. In S. M. Ehrenkranz, E. G. Goldstein, L. Goodman, & J. Seinfeld (Eds.), *Clinical social work with maltreated children and their families: An introduction to practice* (pp. 38–61). New York: New York University Press.

Mishne, J. (1993). *The evolution and application of clinical theory: Perspectives from four psychologies.* New York: Free Press.

Mishne, J. (1996). Therapeutic challenges in clinical work with adolescents. *Clinical Social Work Journal, 24*(2), 137–152.

Mishne, J. (1997). Clinical social work with adolescents. In J. R. Brandell (Ed.), *Theory and practice in clinical social work* (pp. 101–131). New York: Free Press.

Mitchell, S. (1988). *Relational concepts in psychoanalysis.* Cambridge, MA: Harvard University Press.

Mitchell, S. A. (1997, September 20). *New developments in psychoanalytic theory and technique.* Paper presented at the Toronto Institute for Contemporary Psychoanalysis conference, Toronto.

Modell, A. (1984). *Psychoanalysis in a new context.* Madison, CT: International Universities Press.

Montabo, B. (1994). Editorial: A conversation about diversity. *Supervision Bulletin, 2*(1), 2–7.

Moore, B., & Fine, B. (1968). *A glossary of psychoanalytic terms and concepts.* New York: American Psychoanalytic Association.

Morisey, P. G. (1996). Black children in foster care. In S. M. L. Logan, E. M. Freeman, & R. G. McRoy (Eds.), *Social work practice with black families* (pp. 133–147). New York: Longman.

Morrison, A. P. (1989). *Shame: The underside of narcissism.* Hillside, NJ: Analytic Press.

Moss, M. L., Townsend, A., & Tobias, E. (1997). *Immigration is transforming*

New York City. New York: Taub Research Center, Robert F. Wagner Graduate School of Public Service, New York University.

Nagera, H. (1964). On arrest in development, fixation and regression. *Psychoanalytic Study of the Child, 19,* 222–239.

National Urban League. (1979). *Final report: Interagency adoption project.* New York: Author.

Nattusa, J. M., & Friedman, R. J. (1995). *A primer of clinical intersubjectivity.* Northvale, NJ: Jason Aronson.

Neubauer, P. M. D. (1968, May). *Problems of termination in child analysis.* Panel participation at the Annual Meeting of the American Psychoanalytic Association.

Newman, K. (1985, September). *Countertransference: Its role in facilitating the use of the object.* Paper presented at the annual meeting of the Chicago Psychoanalytic Society, Chicago.

Norris, D. M., & Spurlock, J. (1992). Racial and cultural issues impacting on countertransference. In J. R. Brandell (Ed.), *Countertransference in psychotherapy with children and adolescents* (pp. 91–103). Northvale, NJ: Jason Aronson.

Norton, D. (1978). *The dual perspective.* New York: Council on Social Work Education.

Obendorf, C. P. (1954). Selectivity and option for psychiatry. *American Journal of Psychiatry, 110,* 754–758.

Okun, B. F. (1990). *Seeking connections in psychotherapy.* San Francisco: Jossey-Bass.

Olarte, S. W., & Lenz, R. (1984). Learning to do psychoanalytic therapy with inner city populations. *Journal of the American Academy of Psychoanalysis, 12,* 89–99.

O'Neal, V. P., Brown, P. M., & Abadie, T. (1997). Treatment implications with interracial couples. In P. M. Brown & J. S. Shalett (Eds.), *Cross-cultural practice with couples and families* (pp. 15–31). New York: Haworth Press.

Orgel, S. (2000). Letting go: Some thoughts about termination. Plenary presentation—fall meeting of the American Psychoanalytic Association, December 18, 1998. *Journal of the American Psychoanalytic Association, 48(3),* 719–738.

Ornstein, P. (1978). *The search for the self: Selected writings of Heinz Kohut 1950–1978* (Vol. 1). New York: International Universities Press.

Ornstein, P. (1983). Discussions of papers of Drs. Goldberg, Stolorow, and Wallerstein. In J. D. Lichtenberg & S. Kaplan (Eds.), *Reflections on self psychology* (pp. 389–394). Hillsdale, NJ: Analytic Press.

Packer, M. J. (1985). Hermeneutic inquiry in the study of human contact. *American Psychologist, 40(10),* 1081–1093.

Palombo, J. (1985). Depletion states and selfobject disorders. *Clinical Social Work Journal, 13,* 32–49.

Papajohn, J., & Spiegel, J. (1975). *Transactions in families.* San Francisco: Jossey-Bass.

Pedersen, P. B., & Ivey, A. (1993). *Culture-centered counseling and interviewing skills.* Westport, CT: Praeger.

Perez Foster, R. (1993). The social politics of psychoanalysis. *Psychoanalytic Dialogues, 3,* 69–84.

Perez Foster, R. (1996). What is a multi-cultural perspective for psychoanalysis? In R. Perez Foster, M. Moskowitz, & R. A. Javier (Eds.), *Reaching across boundaries of culture and class: Widening the scope of psychotherapy* (pp. 3–20). Northvale, NJ: Jason Aronson.

Perez Foster, R. (1998a). The clinician's cultural countertransference: The psychodynamics of culturally competent practice. *Clinical Social Work Journal, 26*(3), 253–270.

Perez Foster, R. (1998b). *The power of language in the clinical process: Assessing and treating the bilingual person.* Northvale, NJ: Jason Aronson.

Perez Foster, R. (1999). An intersubjective approach to cross-cultural clinical work. *Smith College Studies in Social Work, 69*(2), 269–292.

Perez Foster, R., Moskowitz, M., & Javier, R. A. (Eds.). (1996). *Reaching across boundaries of culture and class: Widening the scope of psychotherapy.* Northvale, NJ: Jason Aronson.

Perlman, F. T. (1997). Psychoanalytic psychotherapy with adults. In J. R. Brandell (Ed.), *Theory and practice in clinical social work* (pp. 202–253). New York: Free Press.

Perlmutter, L. (1996). Using culture and the intersubjective perspective as a resource: A case study of an African-American couple. *Clinical Social Work Journal, 24*(4), 389–401.

Pinderhughes, E. (1982). Afro-American families and the victim system. In M. McGoldrick, J. K. Pearce, & J. Giordano (Eds.), *Ethnicity and family therapy* (pp. 108–122). New York: Guilford Press.

Pinderhughes, E. (1989). *Understanding race, ethnicity and power: Efficacy in clinical practice.* New York: Free Press.

Pinderhughes, E. B. (1979). Teaching empathy in cross-cultural social work. *Social Work, 24,* 312–316.

Pine, F. (1974). On the concept of "borderline" in children: A clinical essay. *Psychoanalytic Study of the Child, 29,* 341–347.

Polombo, J. (1982). The psychology of the self and the termination of treatment. *Clinical Social Work Journal, 10,* 15–27.

Reik, T. (1949). *Listening with the third ear.* New York: Farrar Straus.

Resnick, C., & Dzieglewski, S. F. (1996). The relationship between therapeutic termination and job satisfaction among medical social workers. *Social Work in Health Care, 23*(3), 17–33.

Rinik, O. (1995). The idea of the anonymous analyst and the problem of self-disclosure. *Psychoanalytic Quarterly, 64*(3), 466–495.

Robinson, J. B. (1989). Clinical treatment of black families: Issues and strategies. *Social Work, 37*(8), 323–329.

Robinson, V. (1930). *The changing psychology of social casework.* Chapel Hill: University of North Carolina Press.

Rogler, L. M., Malgady, R. G., Constantino, G., & Blumenthal, R. (1987). What do culturally sensitive mental health services mean? The case of Hispanics. *American Psychologist, 42,* 565–570.

Roland, A. (1996). How universal is the psychoanalytic self? In R. Perez Foster, M. Moskowitz, & R. A. Javier (Eds.), *Reaching across boundaries of culture and class: Widening the scope of psychotherapy* (pp. 71–90). Northvale, NJ: Jason Aronson.

Root, M. (1985). Reaching "other" status: Identity development in biracial individuals. *Women and Therapy, 9*(1), 185–205.

Rosen, H. D., & Frank, J. D. (1962). Negroes in psychotherapy. *American Journal of Psychiatry, 119,* 456 460.

Rotunno, M., & McGoldrick, M. (1982). Italian families. In M. McGoldrick, J. K. Pearce, & J. Giordano (Eds.), *Ethnicity and family therapy* (pp. 340–364). New York: Guilford Press.

Rounds, K. A., Weil, M., & Bishop, K. K. (1994). Practice with culturally diverse families of young children with disabilities. *Families in Society, 26*(3), 253–270.

Rowe, W., Bennett, S., & Atkinson, D. F. (1994). White racial identity models: A critique and alternative proposal. *The Counseling Psychologist, 22,* 120–146.

Ruiz, A. S. (1990). Ethnic identity: Crisis and resolution. *Journal of Multi-Cultural Counseling and Development, 18,* 29–40.

Saari, C. (1991). *The creation of meaning in clinical social work.* New York: Guilford Press.

Saari, C. (1996). Collaboration between psychoanalysis and social work education. In J. Edward & J. B. Sanville (Eds.), *Fostering healing and growth: A psychoanalytic social work approach* (pp. 404–415). Northvale, NJ: Jason Aronson.

Sandler, J. (1976). Countertransference and role responsiveness. *International Review of Psycho-Analysis, 3,* 3–47.

Sandler, J., Kennedy, H., & Tyson, R. L. (1980). *The technique of child psychoanalysis: Discussions with Anna Freud.* Cambridge, MA: Harvard University Press.

Sanville, J. (1987). Theories, therapies, therapists: Their transformations. *Smith College Studies in Social Work, 57,* 75–92.

Sanville, J. (1996). Postlude. In J. Edward & J. B. Sanville (Eds.), *Fostering healing and growth: A psychoanalytic social work approach* (pp. 417–441). Northvale, NJ: Jason Aronson.

Schafer, R. (1973). The termination of brief psychoanalytic psychotherapy. *International Journal of Psychoanalytic Psychotherapy, 11,* 135–148.

Schiff, S. K. (1962). Termination of therapy: Problems in a community psychiatric out-patient clinic. *Archives of General Psychiatry, 6,* 77–82.

Schwaber, E. (1979). On the self within the matrix of analytic theory: Some clinical reflections and recommendations. *International Journal of Psychoanalysis, 60,* 467–479.

Sengupta, S. (2001, March 11). State contract on abuse files is questioned. *The New York Times,* pp. 37–38.

Shane, M., & Shane, E. (1984). The end phase of analysis: Indicators, functions and tasks of termination. *Journal of the American Psychoanalytic Association, 32,* 739–772.

Shane, M. & Shane, E. (1998). Optimal responsiveness and a search for guidelines. In H. Bacall (Ed.), *Optimal responsiveness: How therapists heal their patients* (pp. 75–96). Northvale, NJ: Jason Aronson.

Shannon, B. (1970). Implications of white racism for social work practice. *Social Casework, 51*, 270–276.

Siebold, C. (1991). Termination: When the therapist leaves. *Clinical Social Work Journal, 19*(2), 191–204.

Siebold, C. (1992). Forced termination: Reconsidering theory and technique. *Smith College Studies in Social Work, 63*(1), 325–341.

Sifneos, P. E. (1973). *Short-term psychotherapy and emotional crisis.* Cambridge, MA: Harvard University Press.

Solomon, B. B. (1983). Value issues in working with minority clients. In A. Rosenblatt & D. Waldfogel (Eds.), *Handbook of clinical social work* (pp. 866–886). San Francisco: Jossey-Bass.

Solomon, M. F. (1991). Adults. In H. Jackson (Ed.), *Using self psychology in psychotherapy* (pp. 117–133). Northvale, NJ: Jason Aronson.

Sota, L. (1990). *Working with persons from Asian backgrounds.* Paper presented at the Cross-Cultural Psychotherapy Conference, Hahnemann University, Philadelphia.

Sours, J. A. (1978). The application of child analytic principles to forms of child psychotherapy. In G. Glenn (Ed.), *Child analysis and therapy* (pp. 615–646). New York: Jason Aronson.

Spiegel, J. P. (1976). Cultural aspects of transference and countertransference revisited. *Journal of the American Academy of Psychoanalysis, 4*, 447–467.

Spurlock, J. (1985). Assessment and therapeutic intervention of black children. *Journal of the American Academy of Child Psychiatry, 24*, 168–174.

Spurlock, J., & Cohen, R. (1969). Should the poor get none? *Journal of the American Academy of Child Psychiatry, 8*, 16–35.

Staples, R. (1978). *The black family: Essays and studies* (2nd ed.). Belmont, CA: Wadsworth.

Sterba, R. (1934). The fate of the ego in analytic therapy. *International Journal of Psychoanalysis, 52*, 375–382.

Stikes, S. (1972). Culturally specific counseling: The black client. *Journal of Non-White Concerns, 1*, 55–62.

Stolorow, R. D. (1994). Subjectivity and self psychology. In R. D. Stolorow, G. E. Atwood, & B. Brandchaft (Eds.), *The intersubjective perspective* (pp. 31–39). Northvale, NJ: Jason Aronson.

Stolorow, R. D., & Atwood, G. E. (1992). *Contexts of being: The intersubjective foundations of psychological life.* Hillsdale, NJ: Analytic Press.

Stolorow, R. D., Atwood, G. E., & Brandchaft, B. (Eds.). (1994). *The intersubjective perspective.* Northvale, NJ: Jason Aronson.

Stolorow, R., Brandchaft, B., & Atwood, G. E. (1987). *Psychoanalytic treatment: An intersubjective approach.* Hillsdale, NJ: Analytic Press.

Stolorow, R., Brandchaft, B., Atwood, G. E., & Lachmann, F. M. (1987). Transference: The organization of experience. In R. Stolorow, B. Brandchaft, &

G. E. Atwood, *Psychoanalytic treatment: An intersubjective approach* (pp. 28–46). Hillsdale, NJ: Analytic Press.

Stone, E. (1988). *Black sheep and kissing cousins: How our family stories shape us.* New York: Penguin Books.

Strean, H. (1996). Applying psychoanalytic principles to social work practice: An historic review. In J. Edward & J. Sanville (Eds.), *Fostering healing and growth: A psychoanalytic social work approach* (pp. 1–22). Northvale, NJ: Jason Aronson.

Sue, D. W. (1981a). *Counseling the culturally different: Theory and practice.* New York: Wiley.

Sue, D. W. (1981b). Evaluating process variables in cross-cultural counseling and psychotherapy. In A. J. Marsello & P. B. Pedersen (Eds.), *Cross-cultural counseling and psychotherapy.* New York: Pergamon.

Sue, D. W., & Sue, D. (1990). *Counseling the culturally different* (2nd ed.). New York: Wiley.

Sue, D. W., & Sue, D. (1999). *Counseling the culturally different: Theory and practice* (3rd ed.). New York: Wiley.

Sue, S. (1988). Psychotherapist services for ethnic minorities. *American Psychologist, 43,* 301–308.

Sue, S., & Zane, N. (1987). The role of culture and cultural techniques in psychotherapy: A critique and reformulation. *American Psychologist, 42*(1), 37–45.

Tang, N. M., & Gardner, J. (1999). Race, culture and psychotherapy: Transference to minority therapists. *Psychoanalytic Quarterly, 68,* 1–20.

Tatum, B. D. (1992). Talking about race, learning about racism: The application of racial identity development theory in the classroom. *Harvard Educational Review, 62*(1), 1–24.

Teichner, V., Cadden, J. J., & Berry, G. W. (1981). The Puerto Rican patient. *Journal of the American Academy of Psychoanalysis, 9,* 277–289.

Thomas, A. (1962). Pseudo-transference reactions due to cultural stereotyping. *American Journal of Orthopsychiatry, 32,* 894–900.

Thompson, C. L. (1989). Psychoanalytic psychotherapy with inner city patients. *Journal of Contemporary Psychotherapy, 29,* 137–148.

Thompson, C. L. (1996). The African-American patient in psychodynamic treatment. In R. Perez Foster, M. Moskowitz, & R. A. Javier (Eds.), *Reaching across boundaries of culture and class: Widening the scope of psychotherapy* (pp. 115–142). Northvale, NJ: Jason Aronson.

Thompson, S. (1995). Self-definition by opposition: A consequence of minority status. *Psychoanalytic Psychology, 12*(4), 533–545.

Tolpin, M. (1978). Selfobjects and oedipal objects: A crucial developmental distinction. *Psychoanalytic Study of the Child, 33,* 167–184.

Tolpin, P. (1980). The borderline personality: Its makeup and analyzability. In A. Goldberg (Ed.), *Advances in self psychology* (pp. 299–316). New York: International Universities Press.

Tolpin, M. (1983). Corrective emotional experience: A self psychology revolution. In A. Goldberg (Ed.), *The future of psychoanalysis* (pp. 363–380). New York: International Universities Press.

Toupin, E. (1980). Counseling Asians: Psychotherapy in the context of racism and Asian-American history. *American Journal of Orthopsychiatry, 50*(1), 76–86.

Trop, J. L. (1994). Self psychology and intersubjective theory. In R. D. Stolorow, G. E. Atwood, & B. Brandchaft (Eds.), *The intersubjective perspective* (pp. 77–93). Northvale, NJ: Jason Aronson.

Tyson, P. (1978). Transference and developmental issues in the analysis of a pre-latency child. *Psychoanalytic Study of the Child, 33*, 213–236.

Tyson, P. (1980). The gender of the analyst in relation to transference and countertransference in pre-latency children. *Psychoanalytic Study of the Child, 35*, 321–338.

Vargas, L. A., & Koss-Chioino, J. D. (1992). *Working with culture.* San Francisco: Jossey-Bass.

Vargas, L. A., & Willis, S. P. (1994). New directions in the treatment of ethnic minority children and adolescents. *Journal of Clinical Child Psychology, 23*, 2–4.

Vontress, C. E. (1971). Racial differences: Impediments to rapport. *Journal of Counseling Psychology, 18*, 4–13.

Vygotsky, L. S. (1978). *Mind in society: The development of higher psychological processes.* Cambridge, MA: Harvard University Press.

Vygotsky, L. S. (1986). *Thought and language.* Cambridge, MA: MIT Press.

Walsh, F. (1998). *Strengthening family resilience.* New York: Guilford Press.

Ware, J. C., & Levy, A. (1996). Communities under fire: Empowering families and children in the aftermath of homicide. *Clinical Social Work Journal, 24*, 403–414.

Watts-Jones, D. (1980). Towards a stress scale for African-American women. *Psychology of Women Quarterly, 14*, 271–275.

Wayne, J., & Avery, N. (1979). Activities as a tool for group termination. *Social Work, 24*, 58–62.

Webb, N. B. (1985). A crisis intervention perspective on the termination process. *Clinical Social Work Journal, 13*(4), 329–340.

Weiss, S. (1972). Some thoughts and clinical vignettes on translocation of an analytic practice. *International Journal of Psychoanalysis, 53*, 505–513.

Weiss, S. (1991). Vicissitudes of termination: Transferences and countertransferences. In A. G. Schmukler (Ed.), *Saying goodbye: A casebook of termination in child and adolescent analysis* (pp. 265–284). Hillsdale, NJ: Analytic Press.

Williams, A. L. (1996). Skin color in psychotherapy. In R. M. Perez Foster, M. Moskowitz, & R. A. Javier (Eds.), *Reaching across boundaries of culture and class: Widening the scope of psychoanalysis* (pp. 211–224). Northvale, NJ: Jason Aronson.

Williams, L. F. (1990). Working with the black poor: Implications for effective theoretical and practice approaches. In S. M. L. Logan, E. M. Freeman, &

R. G. McRoy (Eds.), *Social work practice with black families: A culturally specific perspective* (pp. 169–192). New York: Longman.

Willie, C. V., Kramer, B., & Brown, B. (Eds.). (1973). *Racism and mental health.* Pittsburgh, PA: University of Pittsburgh Press.

Wu, D. (1987). *Achieving intra-cultural and inter-cultural understanding in psychotherapy with Asian-Americans.* Paper presented at the Interactive Forum on Transference and Empathy in Psychotherapy with Asian-Americans, Boston.

Zayas, L. H., Torres, L. R., Malcolm, J., & DesRosios, F. S. (1996). Clinicians' definitions of ethnically sensitive therapy. *Professional Psychology: Research and Practice, 275,* 78–82.

Zetzel, E. R. (1956). Correct concepts of transference. *International Journal of Psychoanalysis, 37,* 369–378.

Zimmerman, J. E., & Sodowsky, G. R. (1993). Influence of acculturation on Mexican-American drinking practices: Implications for counseling. *Journal of Multi-Cultural Counseling and Development, 21,* 22–35.

Index

Therapeutic errors
  color-blindness, 25–26, 168
  exclusive focus on ethnicity, 26
  families more different than alike
    perspective, 26
  ignoring cultural focus, 25
Therapeutic nihilism, 24
Therapists. *See also*
    Countertransference
  and anthropological/sociological
    questions, 34–35
  authenticity, 89
  and burnout, 115, 117
  and culturally sensitive training, 28
  demographics of, 24
  and discussion of cross-cultural
    experience, 66
  "dogma and myth" of anonymity, 109
  interpersonal interactional role, 109
  and resistance, 117
    reaction to, 115
  self-awareness and self-observation, 87
  and self-disclosure with patients, 89–90
Therapy, as a two-person interpersonal
    process, 88
Tolpin, Marian, 108
Training programs
  and culturally responsive clinical
    practices, 28–29, 35–36
  questions about, 33
Transference, 32. *See also*
    Countertransference
  case example (American-born
    Hispanic woman)
    cultural identity issues, 100–102
    development/family/psychosocial
      history, 96–100
    ethnic/cultural issues, 102–107
    idealizing transference, 107
  cultural and working through, 183–
    186
  ethnic/cultural/racial transference
    phenomena, 82–86, 95
    "racial transference," 83
    range of responses, 102–103
  hierarchical, 83

  intersubjective view of, 81–82
  modifications in work with children/
    adolescents, 78–81
    "externalization" forms, 80
    problematic adolescent
      transference phenomena, 81
    subtypes of transference, 79–80
  multiple functions of, 186
  narcissistic, 134
  overview (adult clients), 76–77
  resolution at termination, 213
  and self-disclosure, 89–90
  self psychology/archaic selfobject
    transference, 77
Transmuting internalization process, 78
Treatability, 87
Treatment choices
  cognitive behavioral model, 182
  crisis intervention model, 182
  and goals, 182–183
  insight-directed treatment, 47–48,
    75–76
    and stereotypes, 118
  integration of psychotherapeutic
    techniques, 237–238
  short-term dynamic psychotherapy, 117
  supportive therapy, 47, 75, 109–110
Treatment process, 108
Treatment process (beginning phase),
    41–43. *See also* Assessment
    and diagnosis; Engagement
    process; Referral process;
    Therapeutic alliance
  case example (biracial preschooler
    and parents), 57–59
    assessment, 59–60
    ethnic/cultural issues, 60–63
  case example (Puerto Rican
    adolescent), 48–53
    assessment, 53–54
    ethnic/cultural issues, 54–56
  initial interview, 42
    premature conclusions risk, 43
  "optimal responsiveness," 43
  specific issues of culturally diverse
    patients, 39–41